Principles of Practice Management

In Primary Care

Principles
of Practice
Management

In Primary
Care

Edited by
Wesley Fabb & John Fry

This publication has been prepared with the assistance of members of the Standing Committee on Practice Management of the World Organization of National Colleges, Academies and Academic Associations of General Practitioners/Family Physicians (WONCA).

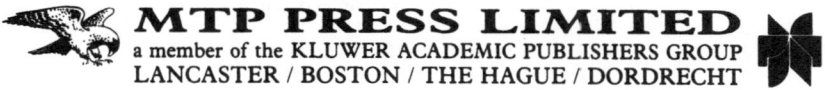

MTP PRESS LIMITED
a member of the KLUWER ACADEMIC PUBLISHERS GROUP
LANCASTER / BOSTON / THE HAGUE / DORDRECHT

Published in the UK and Europe by
MTP Press Limited
Falcon House
Lancaster, England

British Library Cataloguing in Publication Data

Principles of practice management in primary care.
1. Medical officers–Great Britain–
Management   2. Family medicine–Great Britain
I. Fabb, W.E.   II. Fry, John, *1922*–
362.1'72'068   R728

Published in the USA by
MTP Press
a division of Kluwer Boston Inc
190 Old Derby Street
Hingham, MA 02043, USA

Library of Congress Cataloging in Publication Data

Main entry under title:
Principles of practice management in primary care.
    Includes bibliographies and index.
    1. Family medicine–Practice.   2. Medical care.
I. Fabb, Wesley E. II. Fry, John.   [DNLM: 1. Family
Practice–organization.   2. Practice Management, Medical,
3. Primary Health Care–organization & administration.
W 89 P957]
R729.5.G4P738   1984   610   84–7917

ISBN-13:978-94-011-6733-8   e-ISBN-13:978-94-011-6731-4
DOI:10.1007/978-94-011-6731-4

by Butler & Tanner Limited, Frome and London

Contents

Preface

One of the few real and lasting benefits of international medical meetings is the opportunity to meet, talk, gossip and get to know colleagues from other countries.

So it was that we met, talked and planned at WONCA (World Organization of National Colleges and Academies and Academic Associations of General Practitioners/Family Physicians) meetings at Montreux and New Orleans. We realized that although we worked in different places and in different practices 'primary health care' was essentially the same the world over. Our roles, our problems, our clinical content, our challenges and objectives were similar whether we work in Europe, North America, Australasia, South Africa or developing countries.

With such similarities we asked ourselves – 'why not share our common experiences for mutual benefits?' The question developed into an idea and the idea into this book.

We started by selecting what we considered were important topics and then we invited friends and colleagues to join us in putting our experiences and beliefs from years of practice to readers from all over the world to demonstrate our common concerns and to learn from one another.

Intentionally we excluded detailed clinical care. The book is about principles of management and we selected the following broad subjects:

> access to health care
> education of patients as well as physicians
> promotion of health and prevention of disease
> relations with other specialties social
>   and nursing, as well as medical
> the health team and how it works
> management of the practice, policies
>   and planning, records and management.

Selecting our co-authors was easy. Whoever we invited at once agreed to collaborate. We thank them for collaborating and for revising and updating many drafts.

We dedicate our book to the hundreds of thousands of our colleagues who are providing primary health care in the world.

We conceived it to demonstrate that within our different systems of health care that there is a commonality of content, problems and needs for the future and that we teach and learn from one another.

Wesley E. Fabb
John Fry
1984

List of Contributors

Selwyn Carson
Past President, Royal New Zealand
  College of General Practitioners
General Practitioner
PO Box 31050
Ilam, Christchurch
NEW ZEALAND

Wesley Fabb
National Director and Director of
  Education
Family Medicine Programme
Royal Australian College of General
  Practitioners
70 Jolimont Street
Jolimont, Victoria, 3002
AUSTRALIA

John Fry
General Practitioner and WHO
  Consultant
138 Croydon Road
Beckenham, Kent BR3 4DG
UNITED KINGDOM

Edward Gawthorn
Chairman, WONCA Standing
  Committee on Practice Management
General Practitioner
5 Althea Place
Doncaster, Victoria, 3108
AUSTRALIA

Robert Hall
Director of Vocational Training, Box
  Hill Hospital
General Practitioner
'Jarocadah'
Mount Pleasant Road
Eltham, Victoria, 3095
AUSTRALIA

B. Leslie Huffman
Past President, American Academy of
  Family Physicians
Past Chairman, WONCA Standing
  Committee on Practice Management
Family Physician
Deepwater Farm
Grand Rapids, Ohio, 43522
UNITED STATES OF AMERICA

Joseph Levenstein
Head, Department of General Practice,
  University of Cape Town
General Practitioner
163 Koeberg Road
Brooklyn, Cape Town 7405
SOUTH AFRICA

Roger Meyrick
General Practitioner
80 Torridon Road,
Catford, London SE6
UNITED KINGDOM

M. K. Rajakumar
Chairman of Council
College of General Practitioners of
  Malaysia
General Practitioner
38 Jalan Loke Yew
Kuala Lumpur
MALAYSIA

John Smith
Medical Superintendent, Day Hospitals
  Organizations, Cape Town
2 Paterson Street
Newlands 7700, Cape Town
SOUTH AFRICA

1
Access to Care

JOHN FRY (UK) AND JOHN SMITH (SOUTH AFRICA)

In this chapter we seek to show:
What is primary health care
What is good primary health care
How it may be applied in practice.

WHAT IS PRIMARY HEALTH CARE?

Levels of health care

Within every system of health care there are certain inevitable and essential levels of care and service, each with its own features, roles and requirements.

Figure 1 depicts these levels of care and administration, and relates them to population sizes (in a developed country).

The four recognizable levels of care are:

Self-care by the individual in the context of his or her family.

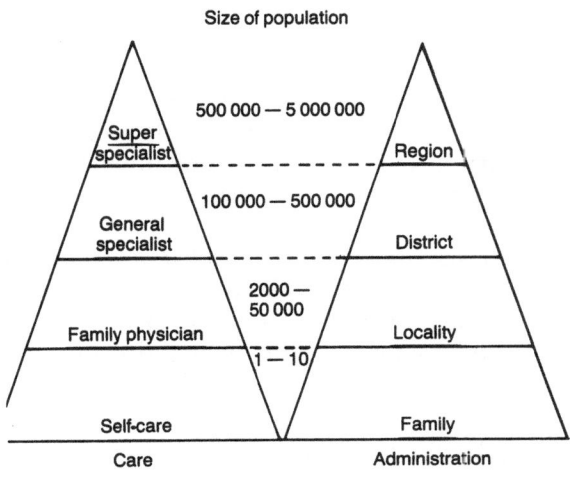

Figure 1   Levels of health care and administration

1

Self-help should apply also to the local community because there are many ways in which community actions will help to improve the health of its inhabitants.

Primary health care by trained workers working within a locality or neighbourhood. These workers may be physicians, nurses, social workers or community health workers.

General specialist care based on a district hospital. This is aimed at providing care by specialist surgeons, physicians, paediatricians, psychiatrists, obstetrician-gynaecologists, anaesthetists and diagnostic specialists as well as visiting specialists from other specialties, for the more common conditions that require hospital care in a district setting.

Sub (or super) specialist care which requires a regional base. It includes the more highly specialized services for the rarer conditions and problems, for example, neurosurgery, chest and heart surgery, and genetic counselling.

Special features of primary health care

There are some *special features* of primary health care that are distinctive to it.

Primary health care services are where *first-contact care* most often takes place. They are where the people should go in the first instance with their problems and diseases. They are where the primary health workers must diagnose and assess these problems, decide on a course of management, and decide whether the condition should be managed at the primary level or be referred to the secondary general specialist or tertiary super-specialist level. As well as first-contact care, primary health care includes *long-term and continuing care* provided by individual doctors, nurses and community health workers for individual patients and families. It is in this process that good long-term relationships are built up between the trained professionals and the people. Primary health care services provide care in *relatively small and static communities*, as distinct from the large, transient and mobile population cared for by hospitals. In developed countries, the population per primary physician (general practitioner or family physician) averages 2500 persons, or even fewer in some countries such as Canada and Australia.

Primary health care has its own *special content of morbidity and mortality* with common minor disorders predominating, these accounting for two-thirds of all consultations, but with chronic diseases making up another one-quarter, and acute major life-threatening diseases and problems one-tenth.

Roles of primary health care workers

Primary health workers, be they physicians, nurses or community health workers have certain roles which they should fulfil. They must be prepared to provide a service for the people. This service should be a personal one, one based on family care and also based on community care.

Primary health care is concerned with preventive and curative care, with rehabilitation and with the promotion of health. Promotion requires education of individual patients and the community (see Chapter 6).

Primary health care workers must function as coordinators of services and resources for the individual patient's good, and be prepared to organize and manipulate the available services. They must be prepared also, at times, to protect the patient from overzealous specialist interventions, and also specialist services from some overdemanding individuals.

PRINCIPLES OF GOOD PRIMARY HEALTH CARE

Good health depends on much more than provision of health services. It depends on considerable self-responsibility and self-help on the part of the individual, and his acceptance and adoption of personal health habits. It depends on social and economic developments that can provide basic social amenities and resources.

Basic good health relies on such undramatic requirements as:

Good mixed foodstuffs
Clean, safe water supply
Public sanitation for disposal of waste and sewage
Child welfare
Maternity care
Family planning services
Prevention of preventable diseases
Control of local endemic disorders
Education of individuals
Education of families
Education of communities
Assessment of the care being provided
Critical self-evaluation of the standards of care and service
Promotion of self-help and responsibility for personal health
Promotion of community involvement and responsibility.

Good primary health care must include the following 'As'. It must be:

Available
Accessible
Affordable
Acceptable
Adaptable
Applicable
Attainable
Appropriate
Assessable

– to meet the needs of the individual, the family, the community and the medical profession.

APPLICATION OF GOOD PRIMARY HEALTH CARE

Having stated some of the general principles of good primary health care, the challenge facing us all is how they can be applied in practice. There are problems and difficulties facing us in developed and developing countries and in affluent and deprived communities.

In *developed countries* our problems are self-made through our self-satisfaction and reluctance to change, or even consider change, in an established pattern of primary care.

The major problem in developed countries is a rigid and historically evolved system of primary health care which has created a medical profession that tends to be inward looking with incentives that are related more to status and money than to service, standards and quality.

In all developed countries there are problems of maldistribution of resources with an inverse relationship to needs. Some areas with high social and economic amenities have too many medical resources which are misused, whilst less affluent and socially more deprived areas have insufficient resources.

In *developing countries* the major problems are poverty, over-population, and inadequate resources which are maldistributed. With more than four-fifths of the population living in scattered rural areas and with four-fifths of the health and medical resources being in the urban cities, such maldistribution results in huge areas and much of the population having no access to health care.

Health priorities in many developing countries have tended to be wrong with too much emphasis on medical technology in specialities and hospitals, and too little emphasis on primary health care and on encouraging community and personal self-care and self-reliance.

Who does what, where, how and why?

In preparing for the future of primary health care it is important that we are flexible enough to consider who should do what? With the evolution of primary care health teams and with the development and progression of primary care workers such as nurse practitioners, medical assistants, feldshers, barefoot doctors, and so on, the role of the physician in primary care must be questioned seriously. That he has a role there is no doubt, but should he continue to perform the same tasks as he does now and has done in the past, or should his training be put to other tasks?

What facilities?

Bearing in mind the nature of primary health care and the roles of primary health care workers, the facilities and resources for good primary health care must be tailored specifically to meet the needs of those seeking primary health care.

There are examples of gross inadequacies in many countries with lack of diagnostic, therapeutic, curative, preventive, rehabilitative and promotive resources. There are examples where there are too many investigations being carried out, too many drugs and other therapies prescribed and too much care being carried out, for the wrong reasons and the wrong incentives.

If access and availability are to be provided, then services have to be fairly organized and distributed and ways discovered of taking good primary health care to the people, even in remote areas.

What planning?

If we are sincere and wish to provide good primary health care for all the people, then some planning controls, directives and evaluations have to be accepted. The challenges are, what plans? what controls? what directives? what evaluation? and for whose good?[1].

What evaluation?

An important issue must be the relevance of the care to the health of the people. Indicators of health and non-health must be defined and used as measures of the progress, efficiency and effectiveness of primary health care. The extent to which the people are helping themselves should also be assessed.

Our current methods and techniques of care and the equipment we use must be the subject of constant critical evaluation. Are they the best ways of achieving stated goals of health and disease prevention and control? Every system of good primary health care must have ongoing methods of data collection by which the qualities of the services provided to the people can be assessed and priorities redefined[2,3].

References

1. Van C. de Groot, H.A., Dommisse, J. and Howland, R.C. (1981). Trends in Obstetric practice at the University of Cape Town, 1967 – 1977. *S. Afr. Med. J.*, **59**, 824

2. Smith, J. (1981). The Day Hospitals organization. *S. Afr. Med. J.*, **59**, 609

3. Smith, J. (1983). *Common Dilemmas in Family Medicine*. p. 211. (Lancaster: MTP Press)

2
The Health Team

SELWYN CARSON (NEW ZEALAND) AND EDWARD GAWTHORN
(AUSTRALIA)

Throughout the world definitions of family/general practice contain phrases like *'family care'* and *'continuous, ongoing, comprehensive care'*. At the same time, with the progressive development of technical skills, there is increasing fragmentation of services and an increasing number of agencies which offer their particular 'thing' to the community. Often there is duplication of services; there is no coordination and most agencies make no commitment and have no responsibility for a comprehensive health service. Along with these developments is the appearance of 'lock-up' general practices where a doctor may live far away from the practice area, commute to work, open the 'shop' from 9 a.m. – 5 p.m. on weekdays and make no house calls. To meet the gap, emergency and crisis services are being created, usually for the transport of patients to base hospitals where diagnosis and treatment is, hopefully, provided. It is not only the victims of motor vehicle accidents and catastrophic life-threatening conditions that are being taken to hospital, but also people with remediable breathing difficulties or chest or abdominal pain, or even minor conditions such as sore throat and ear infections. The accident and emergency departments take on the look of a general practice. The doctors are usually inexperienced in this kind of work and have nothing more than a transient relationship with the patient.

It is not enough for the family doctor to merely be available where other uncoordinated specialist services leave off. It is still possible for him to be generally trained and to keep abreast of the technology, much of which is simple. The GP needs to decide himself what is his job, whether he will provide a 9 a.m. – 5 p.m. consultant kind of service, or whether he will meet the challenge and provide primary health care that includes ongoing responsibility and availability in emergencies, as well as in the prevention of ill-health. If the GP **does** want to stay in the picture, he will have to be trained and equipped for primary health care and, if he should disappear, he will probably have to be reinvented. He is the logical point of entry into a comprehensive health care system. He is aware of what services are available to his patient and able to see that they are delivered. The patient

6

has a right to primary health care that is coordinated and delivered in the local community.

The Todd Report (Royal Commission on Medical Education in UK 1965–68) stated that personal primary health care should be backed by secondary and tertiary care. The total needs of the patient can be anticipated, organized and satisfied, from the stage of prevention to emergency care, after care and terminal care.

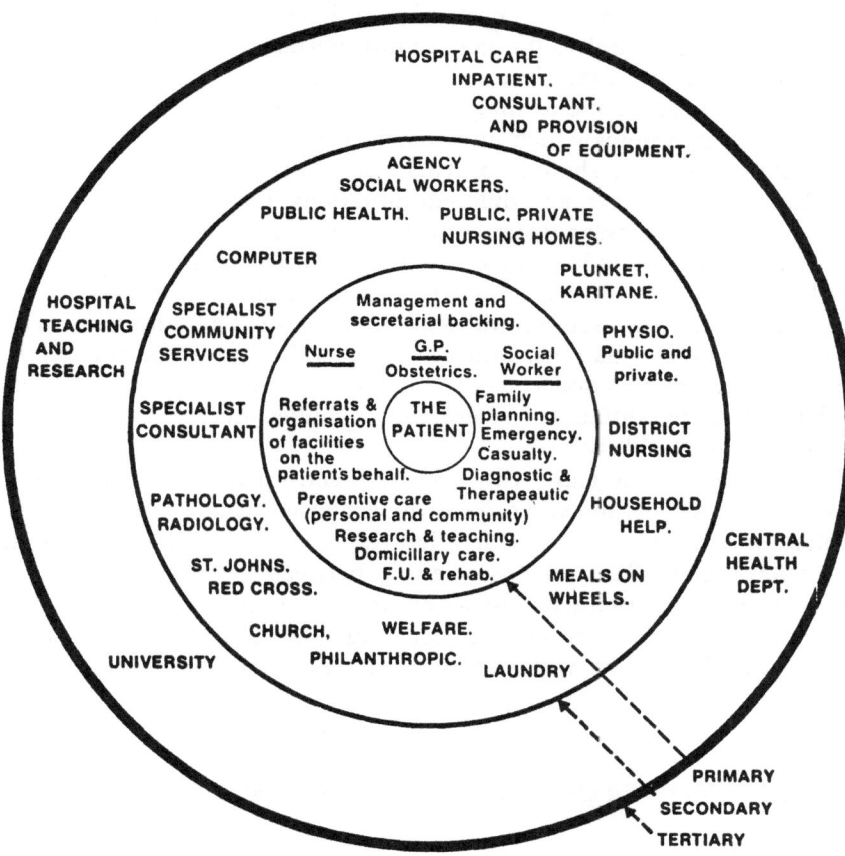

Figure 1 'The Todd Report'

It has been suggested that the conduct of a practice today calls for an investment of equipment and administrative help that can be economically justified if shared by a number of doctors. All over the world the trend has been for doctors to combine into groups. This is a pity in some ways, for the solo practitioner can provide a very good service and often has more opportunity of continuing to provide a personal service. However, the physician does need the help of other professionals to deliver to the community the developing technology. Some physicians prefer to coordinate the team by using a telephone; others find it more suitable to work more closely with the team.

The composition and the size of the health team must depend upon factors such as geography, the community needs, the size of available buildings, the choice of physicians and other members to work solo or in small or large groups, the availability of other health agencies, and the medico-political systems which influence health care. There is no reason why a solo practitioner should not work with a health team.

We have to consider many different situations: for example, the bush nurse linked over a great distance to the hospital or medical back-up, isolated country doctors in neighbouring towns who assist each other, the suburban solo doctor and his wife, the small medical team practice or larger group, and the larger multidisciplinary centre. The same principles apply to all these situations, and *caring for patients* must be the prime objective. Any organization will succeed if this is understood by all team members, and in situations where any member does not meet this objective, failure is likely.

The efficiency of the team will largely depend upon good communications between its members. To have these housed in one building must therefore be advantageous provided that the motivation and organization of the team is good. The loose associations between separate independent and interdependent organizations within the community may operate just as well if good communications and goodwill exist. There may even be an advantage to the patient, with freedom of access to the professionals of his choice.

THE PRACTICE TEAM OF HEALTH PROFESSIONALS

Buildings

If the health professionals are to work together as a team, it is necessary to design a building where they are encouraged to work together. Many health centre buildings have been designed with separation of the health professionals. This encourages isolation. It is necessary also to have some awareness of the services to be provided. If the service is to be comprehensive and include emergency as well as preventive care, the facilities should be adequate.

The building should be easy of access, situated near homes and not in the midst of an industrial area, near the intersection of strategic roads, and near a transport service. Parking facilities need to be available close to the entrance of the building and access into the building should be easy with ramps instead of steps and a wide door to assist the passage of wheelchairs or stretchers. A parmacy in a suitable part of the building and other services can be included depending upon the locality, need and availa-

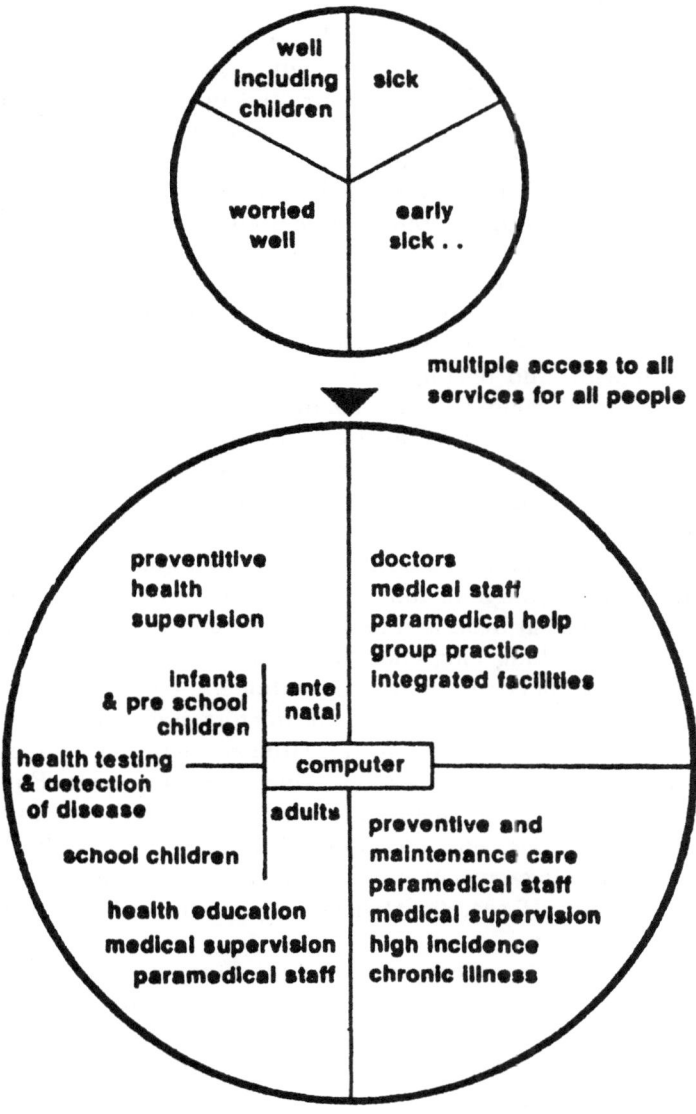

Figure 2   The services in the centre

bility. Passageways in the building should be wide to allow internal traffic, and comfort is as important as cleanliness.

The reception area should be for preference near the entrance and out of sight of anyone waiting, the telephonist must be out of earshot of the waiting and reception area, and the cashier is best situated near the exit and clearly visible. The patients' records storage space should be close to the reception area and the typists are best situated nearby and, ideally, in a room of their own.

If the group is larger than four doctors and their co-workers, two or more smaller waiting areas are better than one large one. Even in a very large centre, it is possible with careful design to give the impression of little movement and traffic if waiting areas are split up and several consulting rooms are grouped around each waiting area. A badly designed building for as little as three or four doctors can give the impression of noise and over-crowding and people being herded about.

The individual consulting rooms can be used by all professionals. Each doctor and co-worker needs a place to keep personal equipment and some centres find that more efficient use of consulting space results if the doctors or others vacate the consulting rooms at the end of each session. A communal work room should be provided where records may be attended to, mail dealt with, and telephone calls made without taking up further expensive consulting room space. A small kitchen, a staff room and toilet facilities should be situated away from the working area and may be combined with a seminar or educational room. There is a lot to be said for all people in the building using the same facilities for relaxation. The best communication can be over morning tea or lunch.

The consulting rooms should be at least 12′ × 10′ (3.65m × 3.04m) and contain equipment enough for most consultations. An examination couch with removable light at head and foot, a sphygmomanometer attached to the wall but with tubing long enough to reach into the room, a desk, a telephone, a small bookcase, shelves for stationery, chairs, a washbasin, a cupboard and a mirror are essential. Some doctors prefer the desk not to be a barrier in the centre of the room but situated against the wall so that there is an open plan or 'sitting room' kind of arrangement. Equipment should include scales for height and weight, a visual acuity chart, equipment for injections, wound cleaning and minor suturing, facilities for the taking of pathology specimens, a vaginal speculum and gloves, and cautery equipment. If secretarial help is available, pocket dictaphone equipment is valuable.

Any accident and emergency area is best situated near the entrance, equipped for the kinds of services it provides, preferably with movable tables or trays, and with a room for minor surgery or larger lacerations equipped with a good light and special table. A cleaning or sterilizing room should be suitably adjacent.

Storage space is needed for equipment and supplies as is a refrigerator for storing vaccines and some drugs. A safe is needed for dangerous drugs

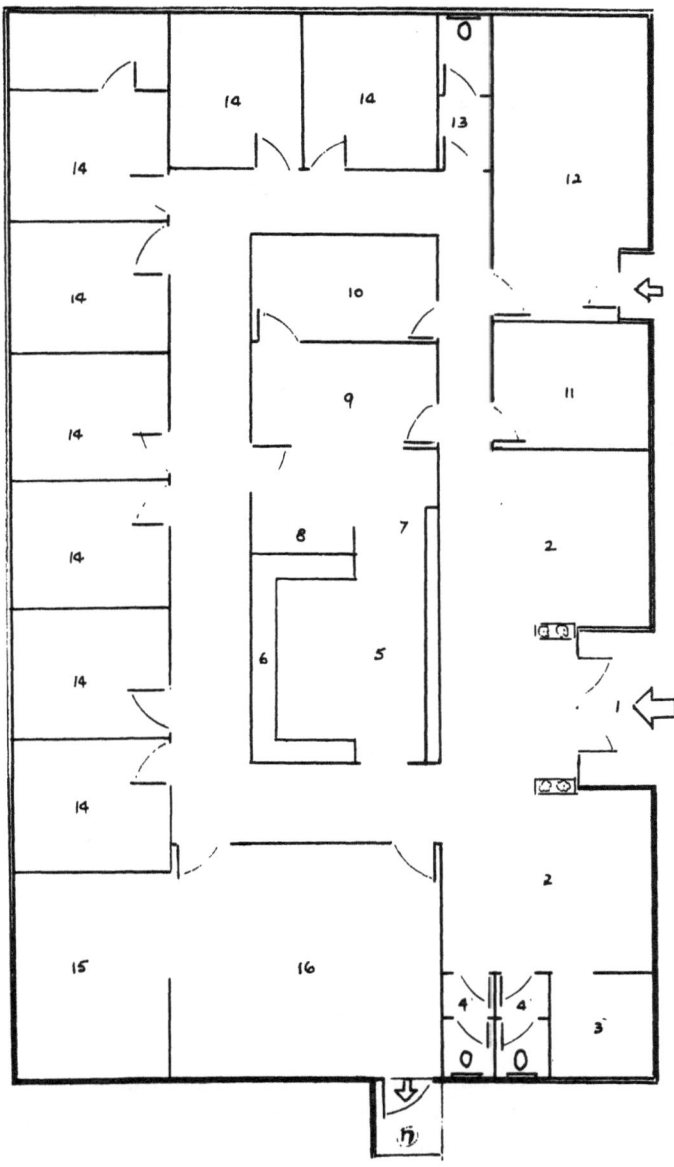

Figure 3   A clinic plan by Dr Edgar Turner

KEY:

1. Entrance	7. Accounts and cashier	13. Staff toilet
2. Waiting area	8. PABX operator	14. Consulting rooms
3. Childrens' area	9. Office manager	15. Treatment room
4. Patients' toilets	10. Typists' room	16. Nurses' area and emergency room
5. Reception area	11. Social worker's room	room
6. Records	12. Staff room	17. Emergency exit for ambulance

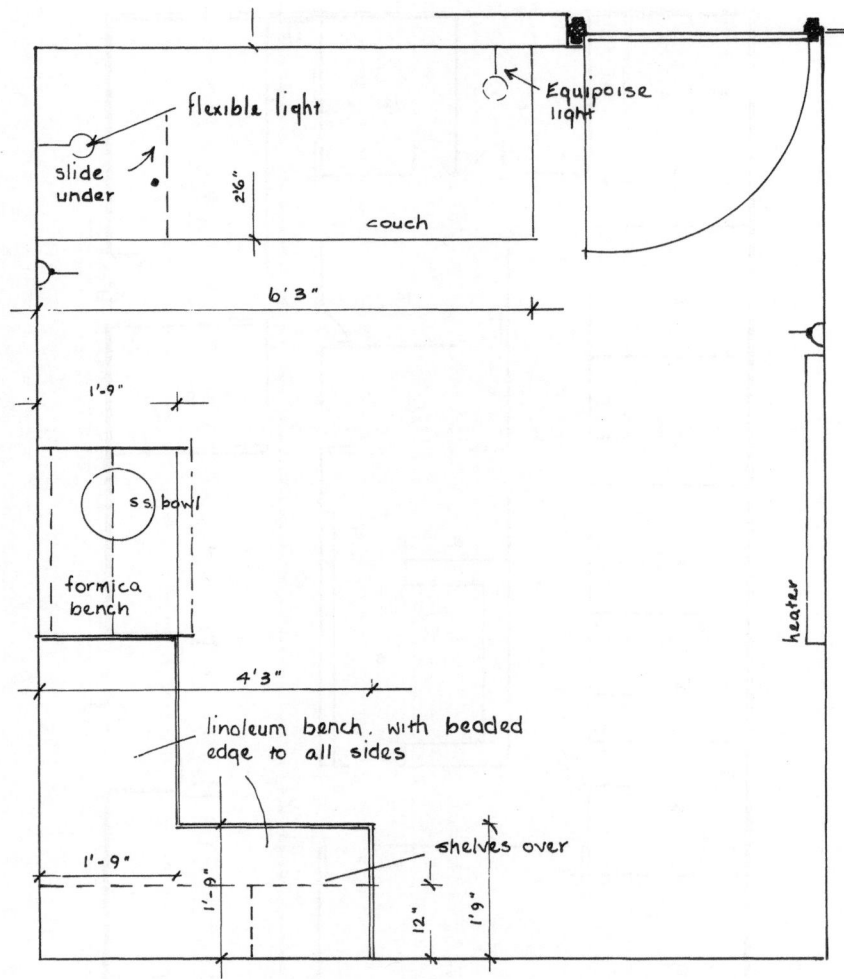

Figure 4   A plan of a consulting room

and cash, and a locked cupboard for other drugs (which can be serviced directly by the local pharmacist). Some centres are large enough to have a pathology area where specimens are obtained.

The doctors

General practice and family doctoring is a service occupation. Doctors have a public and a community responsibility but, above all, they should provide a personal service to the patient. It is possible and very important that, with the inclusion of larger numbers of people in primary health care, a personal service to the patient should be retained. The doctor should be responsible directly to the patient for the work of the team, and part of his training should include the understanding of the roles of other health professionals and the need to work with them. The doctor should be trained as the probable leader and coordinator of the primary health care team. This does not mean dictatorship and direction by the doctor of other health professionals. It does mean the patient has someone to look to for primary health care. As the Balints indicated in their classic research into the relationship between the patient, the GP and the specialist, when more than one professional is responsible for the patient, often no one is finally responsible.

Numbers of doctors

Patients feel, usually, that something may be lost with the development of the larger primary health care centres. The wear and tear on the doctor may be less, but patients find it more difficult to communicate with the doctor and may feel part of a herd of patients. The patient can be heard to say 'I get a different doctor every time.' It **is** possible to do a lot about this problem, beginning with the design of the building. The individual doctor must always be accessible to reasonable communications from the patient. To do this it may be necessary to limit the size of the practice.

There seems to be no absolute ideal number of GPs in any centre and the number will vary from place to place, depending on the needs of the community and the motivation of the doctors. A group of four doctors is a reasonable number for most GPs to work with. A four doctor centre, or groups of four doctors in suites in a larger centre with common staff room and meeting facilities, may be the best compromise. The advantages of the larger groups are that they can afford more equipment, an easier 24 hour coverage, finance for vacations, study leave and sabbaticals and can employ any staff they think they need, such as a practice social worker. In a group that works well, peer review develops inevitably with maintenance and improvement of standards. General practice is a stressful occupation and group support is a major benefit, particularly in situations such as terminal care.

The medical receptionist and secretary

The importance of these team members cannot be overemphasized. Perhaps for too long we have concentrated upon the training of other health professionals and forgotten the role of our support staff. As the first person whom the patient contacts and who is therefore required to judge priorities as well as make the patient welcome, a good receptionist is invaluable. A bad one can be disastrous.

The roles of the receptionist and secretary overlap to some extent and may be combined by one staff member in small practices. However, there are important differences between their respective duties and these will be discussed later. In the study of these roles, let us consider the development of the 'nuclear' health team or family; and indeed, if the patient can see this team as being a family, there is much to encourage him in realizing that a caring relationship exists. One patient, when asked to write down in a few words the definition of a family doctor, stated: 'A qualified, dedicated, member of my family.' Surely the same definition could apply to all members of the team and especially to the receptionist. Consider the following diagram.

The Development of the 'nuclear health' team

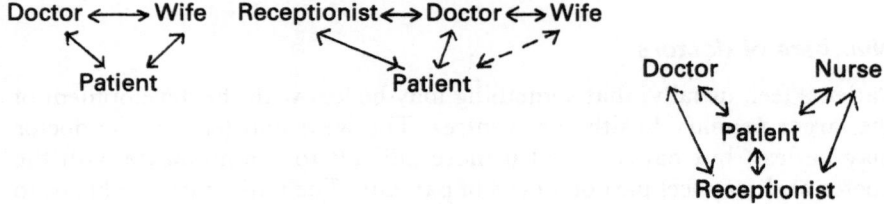

Figure 5   The nuclear health team

The role of the doctor's wife appears to diminish as the modern organization of the group builds up. This can be difficult for the wife to cope with and is a source of one of the difficulties of the medical marriage. A young doctor may start off in a solo practice, perhaps in a country area, and his wife plays an invaluable role in the running of the practice. She can get to know the patients as well as the doctor and be involved in the rich life of the family practice. With the transition to a larger practice, the professional receptionist, secretary, practice nurse and practice social worker take her place and the wife may, quite suddenly, have to face a change of her lifestyle that is very dramatic. The change is probably more important even than that which faces healthy sixty-year old people who have to retire compulsorily from important jobs. The wife will need help to understand that this is not a personal situation and a rejection of her, but rather the inevitable development that occurs when family practice has to be geared to cope with the modern community.

There is some evidence in many countries of a return to solo practice. The roles of its members and their need for efficient communication remain the same. With these concepts stated we may now define the role of a medical receptionist.

What is a medical receptionist?

Everyone knows, or thinks that they know, the answer to this question. But do they really know? The definition is important.

A medical receptionist is a **trained** person. No one, therefore, without such training, should be a medical receptionist. Usually the receptionist is the first person of the health team that the patient meets. Accordingly, she must be properly trained to receive patients and requests for medical services. She should be able to classify patients according to the priorities of their complaints. She must act as an intermediary between the patient and the doctor or other health professionals, ensuring that their work proceeds smoothly and efficiently.

She must be ready to supply necessary information to the patient, to interpret instructions given by the doctor and to make sure that the patient understands what is expected. She must assist in office routines. She must know something of first aid and be prepared to assist patients in emergencies when no other help is available. She must identify herself with the patients' needs and show she cares for the people who attend the clinic.

She ought to have a pleasant personality, an efficient manner, a clean appearance and be sympathetic to the needs of patients.

With each patient seen her duties will normally include the following:

1. Making appointments, either by telephone, or when the patient attends.
2. On reception of the patient, withdrawing from file clinical records, ensuring that all recent X-rays, pathology tests, or other reports required for the consultation are available in correct order, and that the accounts procedure is initiated.
3. Conducting the patient to the doctor's surgery in correct order and with minimum delay.
4. On departure of the patient, writing receipts where appropriate, making advance bookings, ensuring that the patient understands instructions, and correctly filing all records.

In summary, a medical receptionist needs to perform her duties with sympathetic *understanding*, maintaining a *calm manner* and using a high level of *common sense*. Most of her problems can be solved by use of these attributes. Perhaps one should add that she needs eight arms, ten ears, four pairs of legs and six pairs of eyes! We have stated that a receptionist is a **trained** person. What form should this training take?

It is recommended that every junior commencing her duties should be given a handbook containing basic information about her role. This should include an introduction to her role and that of other members of the health team, information on the policy and routine of the clinic in which she is employed, and information about surrounding health services. She should also receive information on the following: the art of public relations, telephone techniques, after hours routine, office management and systems employed, confidentiality, priorities in medicine, the care and sterilization of instruments, and other matters related to the health system and the procedures which it entails.

It is recommended that no receptionist should be considered trained until after approximately one year of on-the-job training, and where possible during that time she should not be left on her own, without back-up. She may have to make important decisions on medical priorities. Should the pale-looking middle-aged man who attends at reception and says that he does not want to bother anyone but has a 'touch of indigestion', be asked to return tomorrow? At all times, and at all levels of training, the receptionist should be taught to look at the patient and to refer the decision on priorities to the doctor if there is the slightest doubt.

During the period of apprenticeship it is recommended that receptionists attend some form of course, and if none is available, it is the doctor's responsibility to ensure that such training is not neglected. Above all, it is important for senior clinic staff to ensure that an adequate *two-way* communication exists between them and the junior receptionist. Too much fear of the status of the doctor may result in a dangerous reticence on the part of junior staff to communicate important information.

The medical secretary

Much of what has been said above also applies to the important role of the secretary. She needs to be the right kind of person, with the same interest in people as the other health professionals. Again, like the others, she should be chosen for personal as well as professional qualities. Also she needs special training for medical work additional to training and experience in general secretarial duties.

In the training of medical secretaries, the course content should include the following:

1. Anatomy, physiology, illnesses, and medical terminology.
2. Medico-legal subjects, such as principles of confidentiality; government and other regulations; the doctor, the patient and the law.
3. Full information on hospitals and other associated health services.
4. Medical record keeping.
5. First aid and priorities in medicine, as for receptionists.
6. Office management and appointment systems.

She should be able to handle dictatyping and other modern aids to secretarial duties, such as photocopiers. It is recommended that training programmes should include one year of on-the-job experience and special courses, assuming previous non-medical secretarial competence.

The medical secretary can be of tremendous assistance to the doctor or other health professionals, provided that her potential is fully realized, and that she is encouraged and allowed to fulfil her role.

The practice nurse

If there is a single solution to the problem of providing primary health care, it is the better utilization of the practice nurse. In all areas, country as well as urban, there is much medical and preventive health technology to be delivered to the people. In urban areas this should be done as far as is possible **in** the local community. The practice nurse is a 'third arm' of the GP and can work with him as no other kind of nurse can do. She has special skills. It is essential for the doctor and the nurse to be able to work together and trust each other, and for the doctor to support the nurse.

In developed countries, it seems there will be soon an over-supply of
doctors. Some general practitioners feel threatened that the practice nurse
will take over much of his work, but there is always so much more to be
done for people. There is always so much more primary health care to be
delivered. Follow-ups of all kinds, routine antenatal care, health surveillance of infants and schoolchildren, early detection and prevention of
emotional illness, alcoholism and obesity, scrupulous routine preventive
maintenance care in high incidence chronic illness, and preventive and
emergency care of all kinds, are best done in family practice. There are
many tasks that need to be followed up and the practice nurse can often do
this better than the doctor. She works better because she works with the
doctor. There will be always more than enough work for the willing GP to
do and the practice nurse can increase his usefulness; it is a matter of
willingness, training and working together in the interests of the people.

Everywhere, attempts are being made to set down precisely what the
practice nurse should do. The truth is that nobody yet knows what she is
able to do, and her role will vary from community to community and
practice to practice. The working together of the physician and the
practice nurse depends, in great measure, on the personalities of both, the
time they have worked together, and the kinds of patients they serve. It
takes a year or 18 months before the patients approach the nurse directly.
They need to get to know her as they need to get to know the doctor, and
any suggestion that nurses may be seconded into practices in the way they
are directed into wards in the public hospital, is best forgotten. If
physicians are to work with practice nurses, it is necessary to define some
of the routine technical procedures that general practitioners use, so that
the nurses may be able to use them. One attempt to do this is *A Manual for
General Practice* (Carson, 1975) which sets out practical routine care of all
kinds. This includes routine antenatal care, surveillance of infants and
children, routine care in high incidence chronic illness, routine follow-ups,
and care in emergencies. The nurse should be a generalist too. Included in
her education should be basic training in counselling and psychotherapy,
family planning, and the techniques of interviewing and listening.

How the practice nurses and doctors work together will vary from centre
to centre. Some physicians opt for a 'pool' of nurses who respond to
requests from the doctors or the patients. Others prefer that the doctor and
the practice nurse should work together with the patients of one doctor's
practice. It is a partnership to provide a personal service to the patient.

It is educational for the doctor to find that once they get to know her the
patients may seek out the nurse or divulge things to her in preference to the
doctor. The longer physicians and practice nurses work together and learn
to respect each other, the greater is the blurring of the boundaries between
their roles.

Like GPs, most practice nurses are probably not suited to the hospital
hierarchical system and are not submissive people. Doctors and nurses
have had hospital training and when they try to work together in general

practice there can be a role conflict. It is as difficult to change the GP into accepting the nurse as a colleague and to make proper use of her training and ability as it is to get the nurse to abandon her role as a subordinate who stands with her hands behind her back waiting for the doctor to tell her what to do. Both need untraining in some ways and yet more training to work together in primary health care. It is desirable that the colleges and academies of general practitioners and family physicians should cooperate with nursing educationalists in providing this training for both the doctors and the nurses.

The practice social worker

Most doctors have no difficulty in developing a useful relationship with social workers and the conjoint effort can be enjoyable and fruitful. However, the social work profession is a young one and their organizations tend to be political in nature rather than academic. Some make the assumption that this new profession should have the respect and political status of the older ones, but there are difficulties in general acceptance of this view. There seems to be no definition of a social worker and no recognized training, no registration and no statutory obligations. Until these things are defined, it is difficult to see how rewards and satisfactions can be identified and planned.

Some countries assist with the employment of practice nurses by payment or subsidy to the management of the local medical or health centre. The advantages are that control is decentralized and efficiency increases, the health professionals have clearer identification as a team and with the local community, and useless professional competition is minimized. The same advantages could accrue from this method of financing practice social workers.

What has to be worked out is the place of social workers in the community and general practice. Practices throughout the world have employed their own social workers and a core of expertise is being accumulated. It seems the service that the general practice can provide is the richer because the social worker is there.

The social worker develops her own communication with any patients who see her, but she should still work with the doctors who support her. Most GPs find social workers in centralized institutions change their positions frequently. It is rare to be able to identify a social worker from a hospital or a government department who has been in the job for more than a few months or a year or two at the most. It is necessary for the practice social worker to stay in the practice, like the GPs, so that all may get to know her. This kind of practice social worker will know she has the full support of the GPs and her work will be correspondingly more effective. She can work alongside the doctors in conjoint and family therapy, and units like the local geriatric unit can do their job better because she works with the doctors. Forman and Fairbairn (Forman and Fairbairn, 1968) pointed out as long ago as 1968 that the social worker in the practice team becomes a personal helper to the patient in a way that an 'outsider' could never do. Ratoff (1973) in the United Kingdom considered, from his own valuable experience, 'that when the social worker is identified with the patient's doctor she is much more acceptable, with the result that she can spot the social problem earlier'. He considered also, as others who are experienced with practice social workers, that the social worker should not be competitive with the GP, but should help make the primary health care unit work, and facilitate the effective mobilization of community resources for the use of the patient. He saw the practice social worker as a personal link between the GP and the district social services.

It is best for the GP and the social worker to select each other, to know each other and develop confidence in each other. GPs do not refer patients to anyone in whom they do not have confidence. The practice social worker gets to know the local community and resources, and the people get to know her and that she works with the doctors and practice nurses. She must be a generalist too and ready to tackle any task where she feels she can help. She should not be above arranging for placement of elderly patients as this is often a rich field for helping people and families, and for psychotherapy and counselling in its best sense. There is a variety of skills amongst the doctors in any centre and these should be shared with the practice social worker. She should attend the weekly clinical meetings which should be general practice orientated. Many doctors have had experience in psychotherapy, so it is not difficult for them to work with the practice social worker in family situations. There should be ongoing education for all professionals in the field. Marital and sexual problems, deviant behaviour, school refusal, and extramarital pregnancies can be anticipated and tackled much better with the help of the social worker, often in conjoint therapy.

Many doctors have had extensive experience of family planning and counselling on contraceptive techniques. Like the family doctor and the practice nurse, the practice social worker should be a generalist and these skills should be imparted to her. Like the GPs and the practice nurses, the practice social worker should know about grief and death. Her loyalty to her practice should be unquestioned. It is not necessary to supervise her work but merely to support her. She may belong to ongoing social worker groups where she can talk about her casework and share her professional experience with other social workers, but she should not have to account to a hierarchy or be supervised by anyone outside the practice.

Multiple access

The patients will get to know the health professionals and they will need to have access to whoever they choose to consult in the first instance.

The office

Office management will be dealt with in another chapter in detail. Solo

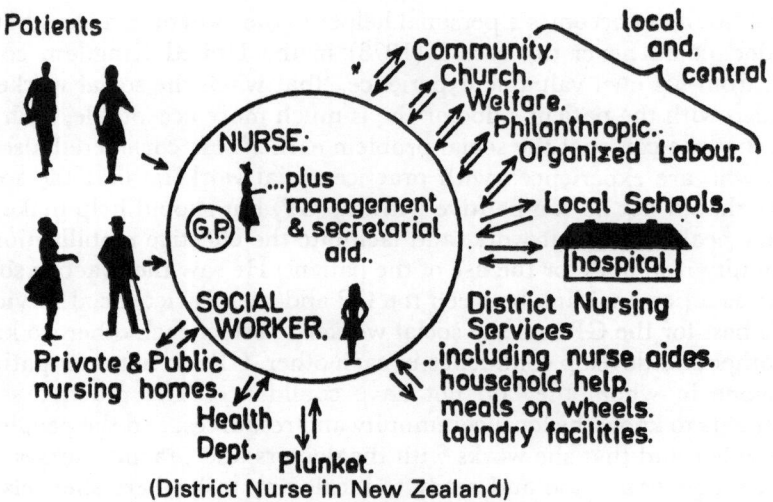

Figure 6   Multiple access for the patient to all professionals

general practitioners work alongside their office and reception areas and are aware of what is happening all the time. This has great advantages. With a large centre and a large staff, the doctors work farther away from the office and are often unaware of what is happening. This is a problem for the patient as communication from the patient to the doctor can be frustrated. From the patients' viewpoint, the reception over the telephone and at the office is as important as anything else that can be provided, and willing and helpful reception sets the keynote for the whole centre.

Practice management is essential and practice management associations in the United States and the practice management committees of the colleges and academies of general practitioners and family physicians have a lot of expertise in all facets of practice management. There is a lot to be learnt from them.

Selection of personnel

The role of the State, government departments and the centralized institutions is to back up the primary health care centres and the keynote should be decentralization as far as is possible. Each centre should be autonomous and competitive and, in those countries where total costs are provided by the State, each centre should be expected to manage its own allocation of funds as far as is possible. The aim of the centre is to treat common illnesses (and this does not mean trivial disorders) in the local community and provide preventive care. In the United Kingdom, the practice team seems to be, most often, not a team but a collection of individuals. This seems to be due to the fact that the members of the team are appointed by their own professional organizations from central offices outside the centres and they are often supervised by them. The differences between this system and that of those countries where centres are able to select and appoint their own staff, including doctors, are dramatically apparent.

The centre should select its own personnel and it should be understood clearly from the outset that all clinical responsibility should remain within the centre. This does not mean that the different professional organizations should not be concerned with the conditions of work, terms of employment and ongoing education of each professional. It means that the staff should be responsible to the centre and all clinical information and allegiance should start and stay in the centre.

Within the centre, the different health professionals should share in the selection of personnel. The senior nurse, for instance, should play a major role in the selection of new practice nurses and, if the habit of the centre is that one practice nurse should work with one doctor, he should also be involved in the selection of the new practice nurse.

Training

The possession of a basic medical degree is a licence to undergo further postgraduate training. The training of family doctors should be done in family practice.

The training of GPs is, at last, becoming very good and training practices are being used all over the world. To have a trainee in the practice is of great value to the centre and it is not acknowledged often enough how much the trainer learns from the situation. The preparation of practice nurses and practice social workers needs a lot of improvement. It is obviously desirable in the future to have student nurses and student social workers involved with medical students in the general practice/family medicine training schemes early in their careers.

Management

Each part of the practice team should have a leader. For example, the practice nurses should have a senior nurse who is paid more for her responsibilities and the office should have a senior person or a manager. Each of these people should be responsible for the administration of their particular part of the team and the nurses or the office staff should be expected to work with, and through, these leaders unless there is an emergency or breakdown in communication. There is nothing more conducive to dissatisfaction than to hear a receptionist say to an office manager, 'But the doctor told me to do it this way'.

It is good management to have 'management group' meetings between the heads of each 'department' (which everyone in the centre will know about). This serves not only as a place for communication between the different parts of the centre, but also demonstrates that the leaders of the office and the nurses are backed up by the others, including the doctors.

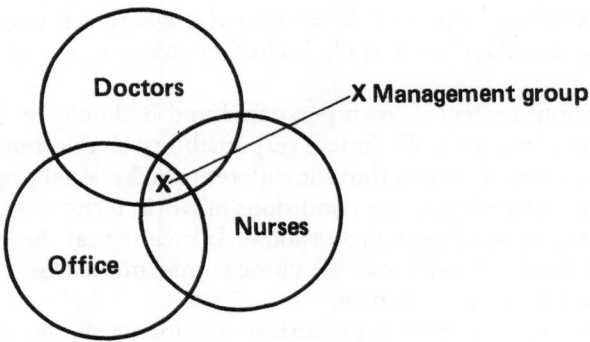

Figure 7   Management group of leaders

Management *amongst the doctors* has its own special problems. There are many examples of GPs who work together happily for many years. There are many other situations where partnerships break up.

It seems that GPs are essentially individualists and possess a rugged, democratic point of view. This is a healthy characteristic when it is used on behalf of the patients, but may cause interpersonal problems in larger groups. Again, four man/woman groups (maybe alongside and in cooperation with other four man/woman groups) seems to be the solution. This seems to be the largest number of doctors who can work together as equal partners without a formal management arrangement. With a larger group, it is wise to keep the central policy-making group down to four members or less. The other doctors can be associates or colleagues or assistants. There should be opportunities for all doctors to discuss money matters or clinical arrangements or staff organization, while the management decisions remain in the hands of the four principals.

There are many ways of sharing income amongst doctors, but basically there are two arrangements. The first is to share the total income after expenses are paid; the second is for the doctor to take what he earns by his own efforts and share expenses with the others. There can be friction if income is shared if there is a feeling that one person does not work as hard as do others. In this situation it is often surprising, when figures are inspected, how little real difference there may be in the income generated by different doctors. The advantage of a shared income situation is that doctors are more often able to agree on reasonable expenditure in buying equipment and developing facilities.

Communications within the centre

Weekly clinical meetings (as distinct from formal case conferences which are necessary when people do not work closely together), and ongoing education are the life-blood of the centre. It is necessary also for the *different* professionals in each centre to have their own small meeting – doctors, nurses, office personnel and so on – to work out their own programmes and how they will work with others.

Records are an important method of communication within the team. They should be typewritten and problem orientated. It is not appreciated generally that to keep good records, which is part of proper patient care, it is often necessary to limit the size of a practice. There is no point in accumulating more patients and responsibilities when one is unable to look after the ones for whom one has taken responsibility already.

Confidentiality is also important when a group of people has access to them. This becomes of great importance when governments begin to develop centralized and computerized medical records. It is obvious that the public hospitals are heading for difficulties here. The solution, in general practice, seems to be to allow the patient to have access to his own records, in the manner of Weed (Weed, 1971), and only what is acceptable to the patient is recorded. Anything discreditable or really confidential should remain unrecorded and between the professional and the patient.

Communication with the patients

There should be easy and pleasant access of patients to the GP or other health professionals. The first job of the GP, practice nurse or practice social worker is to be available when really needed. The telephone system must be suitable for the size of the practice and must not be overwhelmed. There is no point in patients ringing in an emergency if the phone is engaged all the time. There will be improvements in telephone technology, but at present the most commonly used piece of equipment by centres throughout the world is the private automatic branch exchange (PABX) of 12 or 20 lines. It is useful for the patient to be able to dial the same number 24 hours a day and for the call to go through to the professional on duty after office hours. Some practice nurses and social workers are beginning to do their spell of after hours duty just as the GPs do. It is possible to have a commercial answering service connected to the PABX by branch line at night and at the weekends so that it appears to the patient as though the call has been answered by a receptionist in the office. The operator dials the home number of the doctor on duty and plugs the call into it. Answerphones have the disadvantage that the patient has to ring again and this may be difficult in emergencies or when ringing from a call box.

Letters should be typewritten and, more particularly, important medical certificates. A *photocopier*, if it can be afforded, is of tremendous use in communicating details of records to patients, consultants or hospitals, and obviates the need for long and detailed letters.

A blackboard in the entrance to the clinic or centre can transmit messages and there are many opportunities to give printed handouts to patients.

Agreements among the doctors

It is impossible to have agreements to cover every eventuality and legal agreements can work only if there is a spirit of goodwill between all signatories. It is wise to set down basic agreements about employment, associations, liability for expenses, vacations, study leave and sabbaticals, sick leave, dissolution of the practice or association, and the death of partners or colleagues. Where there is expenditure, it should be accounted for. Where the facilities are owned by a minority of the doctors, the valuation for rental purposes should be done by a professional valuer and be available to all.

Agreements with other staff

Practice nurses, practice social workers or practice managers should have security of appointment as do the doctors. The GP should be interested and concerned in the conditions of employment, ongoing education and facilities needed by these professionals.

Problems of the practice team

There is great potential for competitiveness between health workers and much of it may not be for the benefit of the patient, the community or the treasury. Doctors have difficulties in working with other professionals and in recognizing that they have their own skills and may do some things better than doctors in some cases.

The hospital training of doctors and nurses has its disadvantages in the practice of family medicine. It is unpleasant for qualified health professionals to realize that they may have to be 'untrained' a little, and prejudices and preconceptions changed before they can begin to learn again. It is not only medical students who are indoctrinated that general practice is a lower order of service. It happens with nurses as well. One of the attributes of a good GP or a good practice nurse is a willingness to go on learning.

Social workers seem to have their own difficulties and can show great defensiveness if it appears that the GP may be telling them what to do. Like others, they need to accept that it is in the interests of the patient that the GP takes final responsibility for the patient. The social worker and the GP need to be able to communicate and resolve difficulties and the GP, in his turn, needs to know that the practice social worker has her own domain of clinical responsibility. Fortunately, it seems that the eyes of both GPs and social workers are opened when they work together in general practice.

Solo GPs may find it painful to join a group. They may lose the loneliness of working solo, but have to resolve the interpersonal problems of working together with other equal professionals. The solo GP's work comes under scrutiny and his funny, illogical tricks of prescribing are exposed, and this can be embarrassing.

Every now and again, an individual feels he is being exploited or that he is working harder than others. This happens in any group, family or office and it can be salutary for figures to be kept, produced and discussed. Often, it is found that the differences are not as great as were imagined.

It is of value that finance and management should be decentralized as far as is possible in primary health care so that the different workers can know clearly where their allegiances are to be directed. Any team needs acknowledged leadership. This does not mean direction or control at a clinical level, but it does mean that the right people make the decisions. The junior receptionist may make her point of view known but it is not up to her to run the practice. With a team of health professionals it must be clear who is finally responsible for the service of the centre and to whom complaints and dissatisfaction with services should be directed. These principles make for unity in the practice team.

Within the team the problems are the same as in any group. They include jealousies and feelings that occur when work is not being recognized, or when people are not being valued or feel they are being discriminated against. These things are present in any family or group of people. Any leader should be interested in defusing potentially destructive situations and allowing expression of feelings and resolution of difficulties. In general practice, particularly, the art of leadership must also include the humility of being an ordinary member of the clinical team at the right time. As in any family, goodwill and a willingness to get on together is most important.

References

1. *The Royal Commission on Medical Education* (1965–68). London, HMSO
2. Carson, S. (1975). *A Manual for General Practice*, 1st edition, Auckland, Beecham Research Laboratories
3. Forman, S.J. and Fairbairn, E.M. (1968). *Social Casework in General Practice.* London, Nuffield Provincial Hospitals Trust
4. Ratoff, L. (1973). More social work for general practice. *J.R. Coll. Gen. Practit.*, **23**, 736–742
5. Weed, L. (1971). *Medical Records, Medical Education and Patient Care.* Cleveland, Western Reserve

3

Relations with Specialists in Clinical and Allied Health Professions

SELWYN CARSON (NEW ZEALAND)

OTHER GENERAL PRACTITIONERS

The attitude should always be helpful and one should be accessible for communication. Dealings should be ethical and polite even in bad circumstances. Scrupulousness in dealing with another's patients is essential and if, in any emergency, one should see another's patient, it is wise and in the interests of the patient to let the patient's own doctor know the details.

When a patient wishes to change from another doctor and it is likely that there were difficulties between the patient and the person's doctor, ask about it. It is always a good policy to ask the patient to notify the previous doctor of the change and to request a transfer of records. This is an advantage to the patient and to the doctors and one has the advantage of starting with an honest relationship all round. If the patient should present while in active therapy with another, find out why this is happening. It may be that the patient may have had infantile needs mobilized by his relationship with the previous doctor and may not have been able to withstand any confrontation by the other doctor. This may need defining before any change is made, and it may not be in the patient's best interests that another should assume responsibility for therapy at that point. The situation may be a reflection of a difficulty in the patient's personal relationships, and if it is not sorted out, the patient may not just transfer his allegiance, but also his difficulties in relationships.

If you treat other doctors and their wives, by all means roll out the red carpet and give willing service, but come to an arrangement early on that they will have the benefits of the same objective care and good records just as do other patients. If there is anybody who gets less proper care than a sick doctor, it is a doctor's own sick wife.

26

HOSPITALS AND SPECIALIST DEPARTMENTS

Primary health care services need a technical back-up of hospital services and specialists in centralized institutions. It is important that the planning of the central services should start from the primary health care services where the greatest proportion of patient care takes place. Geriatric and psychiatric services, for example, should start in the local community and not in centralized units, if they are to be of real value.

In some countries the GPs have been isolated from the hospitals for many years and are only now beginning to return. Like all large institutions, hospitals tend to take on a life of their own and become disassociated from the needs of the people they are supposed to serve. One cynic remarked that it was the best thing that could have happened to general practice that GPs should have been excluded from the hospitals, for they have had a better opportunity to stay in touch with people and community needs. This may be so, but it is only in the last few years that primary health care has come into its own and the GP's contribution to the hospital has been seen to be of value. In places like Vancouver, the family physician has always had equal rights with other doctors to care for his patients in hospitals and this should be the pattern in other countries. Entry will be mostly through the developing departments of general practice. It is necessary for the people who work in these departments to remain general practitioners with their roots in the community and not become academicians and administrators.

If primary health care is doing its job, the basic relationship with specialist units, base hospitals and centralized services should be as illustrated in Figure 1.

CONSULTANTS

We could not function well without our specialist colleagues. Their special technical expertise can be astounding even to other doctors, but it must be understood that their role is to help the GP to care for his patients when requested and to respond with all their skills when they are needed. Specialists are often our teachers, but they are always our helpers. It is to the patient's advantage that he can look upon the GP as the one who is finally responsible to him and it is up to the GP to support the patient in his dealings with the massive and confusing health system organization. It must be the personal doctor who guides the patient through the medical jungle, with all its potential hazards. When referring a patient to a consultant, do not hesitate to state what you require from him. If you seek only an opinion and the patient not to be treated, then say so and the specialist will not be upset. The skills of specialists in their own fields are so great, and the things they can do for our patients so impressive, that they have no need to take on extras. A good specialist is grateful to get on with his own job and does not want to be the GP. There is nothing sadder

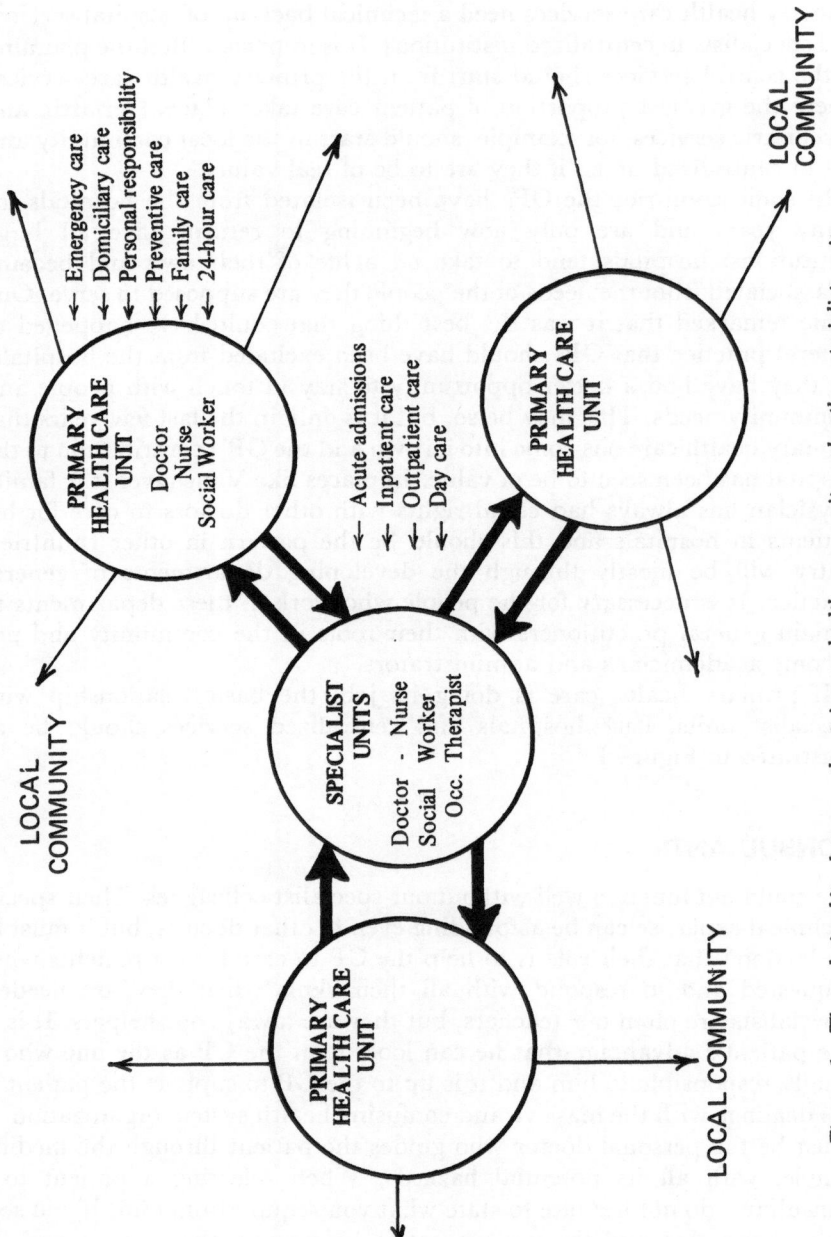

Figure 1 The relationship between the primary health care unit and other specialist units.

and more perplexing than for, say, a gynaecologist to have to prescribe psychotropics.

If there has been an interspecialist or interdepartmental referral for which you have not asked, and which is not acceptable to you, then indicate your feelings about it. Consultants and specialist departments like to know where they stand with you. Be polite and cheerful about it and if you do feel the specialist has been disconcerted by your indicating your feelings, then send him a patient or two as soon as possible to let him know that you enjoy working with him and have respect for his skills!

'OUTSIDE' SOCIAL WORKERS

These are our co-workers and the skills they have must be understood by general practitioners. We must be able to work with them and the social worker must be able also to understand that general practitioners are now trained in counselling and psychotherapy. GPs have a tradition of widely interpreting what should be their personal service and responsibility to patients and often this does not stop at physical diagnosis and the prescribing of drugs.

It is often difficult to be available to social workers on the telephone at all times because there are so many of them associated with different organizations. It is a great advantage to have a practice social worker who can share the load.

PHYSIOTHERAPIST AND OCCUPATIONAL THERAPIST

These are amongst the most useful and reliable of professional colleagues. They work easily with doctors although, like all hospital trained workers, they have had little preparation for working in general practice. Again, it would be beneficial if students in these disciplines were involved early on in training with medical students in general practice. It is necessary to understand their skills and their point of view and accept their opinions.

NURSING SERVICES

It is cumbersome, expensive and an indication of bureaucratic misman-agement that community nursing services have developed without work-ing alongside the GPs, and that the different kinds of nurses working in the community tend to be competitive. It makes sense that the district (community) nurse should work with the practice nurse, the GP and the practice social worker. The roles of the different kinds of nurses are interchangeable in many circumstances and there will be a need in the near future for 'community nurses' to have a broad community-oriented training rather than the traditional hospital one, so that they can carry out a variety of tasks with the general practitioner. Ideally, the nurses should be employed by the local centre even though they have professional links outside the centre. This makes for decentralization and the clear identification of the nurse with the medical centre and the local community.

THE PHARMACIST

Of all our colleagues the pharmacist is amongst the most valuable. He is informed and educated and often acts in the best interests of the doctor as well as the patient. We have all been informed of an error we have made in prescribing by a friendly and alert pharmacist. He is often aware of non-compliance and the possible misuse of drugs, and often has a lot of information which would help both the patient and the doctor. It is wise to include the pharmacist in the centre weekly clinical meetings.

SCHOOL TEACHERS

More communication is needed with school teachers and they need more GP support in their work. The best situation occurs when the local centre is involved in the routine surveillance of children, including school children, as part of the work of the practice. This can be done very easily by the practice team and protocols for this are developed easily. Children should be examined in infancy and before they go to school. The surveillance should be systematic and based on the infant immunization schedule and is best done by the practice team at the local centre.

CLERGY

Like the GP, the clergyman has a special relationship with the patient and relatives in sickness and death and an ongoing communication with families. There can be nobody more useful than the local clergyman, but it is a great disappointment that so many of the clergy have somehow become 'spiritual consultants'. They have not developed the basic skills of counselling and psychotherapy which are learned so easily, and have left whole parts of their practice to other professionals who are emerging in the community. There are signs that the clergy are becoming more aware of their obligations.

LAWYERS

If a lawyer asks for a report from the family doctor, it should be prepared scrupulously and typewritten. A copy should be retained. If a patient says his lawyer requires a report, ask the patient to instruct the lawyer to write to you setting out just what report is needed. The fee should be realistic and compensate for all the time taken in the examination of the patient and the preparation of the report. The account should be sent to the lawyer when the report is sent.

If an opinion is needed about the testamentary capacity of an

E35

The Locum Tenens

The employment of Locum-Tenens implies a contract between the Doctor, the Locum and the Patient for the servicing of the patient's health needs.

(1) Responsibilities of the Principals –
The principal must verify:

1.1. That the Locum is adequately skilled to perform the duties required of him.
1.2. That the locum has a valid Practising Certificate.
1.3. That the locum is a member of the Medical Protection Society or the Medical Defence Union.
1.4. That the locum understands the organization of the Practice/s in which he is employed including the structure of the Practice/s.
1.5. That the locum understands the health care facilities both in the community and in the hospitals of the region. This would include methods of referral to consultants, admission to hospital and co-ordination of activities of associated health professionals to ensure good health care of the patient.
1.6. That the locum understands the terms of employment. A written agreement is preferable.
1.7. That the locum has adequate back-up resources if difficulties arise in the course of his employment.

(2) Responsibilities of the Locum –
The Locum must:

2.1. Fulfil his position and practise medicine in a personal and caring fashion to the best standard of which he is capable in the tradition of the profession in this country.
2.2. Remember that his prime responsibility is to the patient for whose health care (in the widest possible terms) he is responsible.
2.3. In no way undermine the confidence the patient has in his own Doctor.
2.4. Not use the locum position to build up a practice of his own – patients must always be returned to their own Doctor on the expiry of the locum position.

2.5. Not undertake procedures which he is incompetent to perform.
2.6. Not undertake responsibilities and a work load he is unable to cope with.
2.7. Report back, on the completion of the engagement, details of services provided, diagnoses and treatments to ensure continuity of care.

(3) Fees –
Most complaints about locums arise in this area and, therefore, locums must know the range of fees charged by his Principal for particular services. Total fees for a service at a particular time should be established and from these fees the applicable benefits deducted. The requirement that fees be paid before a patient is seen is unacceptable as is the demanding of fees in cash.

(4) Terms of Employment –
It is recommended that locums be employed on terms which give them incentives and adequate monetary returns for their work. They should not be employed unrelieved for unreasonable periods of time. The preferred method of remuneration is that of a salary, plus expenses, plus incentives. If the salary is based on gross earnings, then reasonable practice overheads should be deducted. The practice which has arisen of locums expecting and taking all they earn for a period is to be resisted.

(5) Application of Recommendations –
The above recommendations should apply to individual locums as well as commercial locum services.

Dr John Musgrove

Figure 2 The locum tenens

individual, it is best to conduct the examination in the presence of the lawyer. The important questions to ask include the amount and values of the patient's possessions and what disposition is intended and why. Many a GP has been made to look a fool in a subsequent dispute in court because these pertinent questions were not asked.

POLICE

The police often have unpleasant duties and it is the GP's responsibility to help wherever possible in the interests of the community. In emergencies, the taking of specimens such as blood, and the examination of victims of assault, the GP can be useful. If a policeman requests a home visit for a patient, go immediately. The police have a reputation for being helpful and tactful.

LOCUM SERVICES

If there is a locum employed in the practice then the relationship should be clear. Details of a useful arrangement are to be found in Figure 2.

4
Providing for Emergencies in General Family Practice

JOSEPH LEVENSTEIN (SOUTH AFRICA)

The issue of the handling of the emergency call, and whose responsibility it is, is at the centre of a controversy in several countries throughout the world. With the advent of sophisticated and expensive emergency care delivery systems, the general practitioner has handed management over to emergency care specialists, in some instances gratefully, in others reluctantly, and in most, without much thought.

I believe that an overall policy for the management of emergencies should be instituted, which should take into account contributions from all disciplines and utilize all facilities for the best possible cost–benefit ratio.

An emergency may be defined as any situation which is interpreted by the doctor as requiring immediate attention.

In South Africa, fortunately, the general practitioner's responsibility in an emergency call is clear. The South African Medical and Dental Council firmly state that ' . . . in cases of emergency a practitioner is compelled to render assistance'. This ruling can even be interpreted broadly to mean that a doctor may not deliberately ignore an emergency situation such as a motor car accident. In other countries, the situation may not be as clear-cut.

What skills (attitudinal, knowledge and psychomotor) does the general practitioner require to handle emergencies? Also what equipment, and organizational and practice management arrangements should be instituted to cope with emergencies? Finally, should and can the general practitioner handle emergencies?

SHOULD GENERAL PRACTITIONERS HANDLE THEIR OWN EMERGENCIES?

There are good reasons why a general practitioner should handle emergencies in his own patients as part of their continuing care. He has prior knowledge of their illnesses and behaviour and is therefore in the best position to meet the patients' physical and psychological needs in an emergency situation. He also knows which of his patients are at special risk. As he usually serves a circumscribed area and has knowledge of the local geography, he can render his services *promptly*. Also, as he is part of the existing medical structure, his services can be provided at no extra cost to the community. The general practitioner has a most important function to perform in predicting and preventing emergencies. As a result of his unique relationship with his patients, he can educate them according to their own individual needs. If, for example, he accepts that every 'unexpected' status asthmaticus, acute heart attack or suicide bid could be regarded as a therapeutic failure, and if he investigates what could have been done to prevent these – for example, did he ignore warning signs, or did he educate patients to report deviations from their norms? – then, by this self-audit he may go a long way towards the possible prevention of further emergency situations in his practice.

The general practitioner should use every opportunity for patient education. Should we not display in our waiting rooms 'buckle up' for example? His educational responsibilities should also extend to the training of ambulance men and first aid men.

In arguing against the general practitioner continuing his traditional function of treating emergencies, there are those that maintain that emergency care is too disruptive of modern day family practice. There are no hard data to support this claim. In fact in the commonest and most important emergency of all, acute myocardial infarction, it was shown in the Cape General Practitioner Coronary Care Project, that in line with other Western countries, most participating general practitioners did not receive more than twelve calls per year. Of the 119 participants who completed the questionnaire, after the project was completed, 71% stated that the policy of an *immediate* response to all suspected cases of acute myocardial infarction had only 'negligibly' disrupted, while 10% thought their practices had been 'grossly' disrupted. (In fact this survey showed that general practitioners were at least as effective as mobile intensive coronary care units in the prehospital management of myocardial infarction.)

Information from morbidity surveys indicates that there are only one to ten emergency calls per month, many of these occurring after hours, and consequently not disruptive of the practice routines.

TYPES OF EMERGENCIES

1. Chest pain
2. Respiratory distress
3. Severe haemorrhage or dehydration
4. Debilitating pain
5. Multiple injury
6. Any psychiatric condition which can result in destruction, or harm to self or others

7. Poisonings
8. Sudden loss of consciousness
9. Convulsions (under certain circumstances)
10. Severe allergic reactions
11. Shock-like states not already mentioned, as in septicaemia
12. Any other problem requiring immediate attention.

KNOWLEDGE

This list in fact comprises the conditions of which a general practitioner should exhibit adequate knowledge in the area of emergency care. He should know the natural history of diseases causing such symptoms or signs, and the drugs and equipment needed to treat them.

PSYCHOMOTOR SKILLS

In handling an emergency, the general practitioner should have mastered the following skills;

the eliciting of physical signs and the assessment of the clinical condition of the patient

intravenous fluid administration

cardiopulmonary resuscitation

splinting and other first aid procedures

positioning and moving of patients

maintenance of respiration, and use of the Ambubag, oropharyngeal tube and endotracheal tube

catheterization

performance of ECGs

trochar and cannula insertion

stomach washout

minor surgical procedures, e.g. suturing.

ATTITUDES

The general practitioner should be aware that in this situation, in the majority of emergencies, he would be authoritarian, calm, reassuring and controlling, and that in this situation he would have a highly dependant patient. He should show awareness of his own limitations. He should be able to liaise effectively and politely with all paramedical and official personnel, as well as his specialist colleagues.

EQUIPMENT AND DRUGS NEEDED

It is thought that these should be divided into groups in separate bags. The lists below contain equipment general practitioners should ideally have. However, certain pieces of equipment would be obtained by the general practitioner only if he had the skills to use them, e.g. a laryngo-scope.

Diagnostic bag

The usual equipment is a stethoscope, ophthalmoscope, auriscope with ear and nose attachments, knee hammer, disposable gloves and chemical sticks (to estimate the presence of sugar in blood and urine, for example).

Bag for parenteral drugs

There are endless sets of drug lists that could be given, and I have confined myself to the following suggestions. Drugs are listed under system or condition headings, and while certain drugs could be used for several systems, they are listed only once.

Drugs

Cardiac

digitalis preparation, e.g. digoxin, oubain
diuretic, e.g. furosemide
lignocaine
atropine
other appropriate antidysrhythmic drugs, e.g. propanolol, verapamil
isoprenaline

Respiratory system

β_2 stimulants
theophylline derivative
adrenaline

Anaphylaxis

steroids
promethazine
adrenaline

Analgesia

morphine or morphine derivative
synthetic morphine or non-narcotic analgesic
antispasmodic
inhalation analgesic

Sedative/antiemetic/anticonvulsant

tricyclic derivative, e.g. chlorpromazine
benzodiazepine derivative
metoclopramide

Miscellaneous

50% dextrose or glucagon
insulin
sodium bicarbonate
blood pressure depressor
ergometrine
syrup of ipecacuanha

Trauma bag

disposable syringes, needles
drip-giving sets, 'butterflies', braunulas (intracatheters)
swabs, bandages, cotton wool etc.
suture and other instruments
splints and other first aid material
fluid replacements
cut down set
trochar and cannula
Ambubag or respiratory assistance equipment
oxygen
laryngoscope
endotracheal tube
ECG machine
suckers
stomach washout equipment.

The general practitioner should check his bags regularly to make sure that drugs are replaced, that they are not out of date, and to ensure that equipment is functional.

PRACTICE MANAGEMENT ARRANGEMENTS

To facilitate prompt and efficient handling of an emergency, the general practitioner should ensure that he is able to be contacted or alerted to one. This entails educating his receptionist to discern which call is a true emergency during consulting hours, and using an effective way (e.g. radio or 'bleep' system) to be called after hours. These arrangements may be included in any off duty roster system with one's colleagues or partners.

Within the practice, it is useful to have lists of those at risk for medical emergencies, for example, coronary artery disease patients, depressives, and patients with chronic respiratory disease. As mentioned earlier, these patients should be educated to report early deviations from their norm, and the doctor should have the appropriate skills to detect these as well. Thereby, it may be possible to prevent many emergencies.

Further education of individual patients could include telling them of, or providing literature on, what constitutes an emergency.

This chapter has been written from the veiwpoint of a general practitioner in active practice who handles the immediate treatment of all his emergencies, in the belief that this is part of continuing care, and that this is the most cost-effective way to deliver this care.

5
Promoting Health – Practice and Principles

ROBERT HALL (AUSTRALIA) ASSISTED BY WESTON ALLEN, RUSSELL
GIBBS, STEWART KINGMA, ROBERT PIGGOTT AND MEMBERS OF THE
PREVENTIVE AND COMMUNITY MEDICINE COMMITTEES OF THE ROYAL
AUSTRALIAN COLLEGE OF GENERAL PRACTITIONERS

SUMMARY

In this chapter, I describe some innovative approaches which have been
applied successfully to promoting health in primary care practice around
the world, and make specific suggestions to enable general practitioners to
incorporate them. The individualistic approaches from industrialized
countries may be more familiar to many readers. Community based
approaches are also outlined, with a summary of the management steps
found effective in developing a participatory community health programme.

INTRODUCTION

Since health practices and sickness care are inextricably bound in the local
cultural patterns of different social and economic structures, it is impossible to write any universally applicable guide to practice management to
promote health and preventive care. Thus I wish to make explicit my
biases. I write as a white Anglo-Saxon Protestant general practitioner with
a liberal humanitarian perspective, mainly to 'first-world' colleagues who
practise in countries with a well-developed productive industrial base
which allows sufficient surpluses to fund nutritional food for all, housing,
and a wide range of human services, including public health measures,
along with personal sickness care. It is mainly to the personal sickness care
providers that I am writing.

Potential roles for general practitioners in health promotion activity
include:

Current activity
1. Routine consulting, including home visiting.

2.   Immunization.
3.   Annual check-ups.
Extended activity
4.   Health risk assessment.
5.   Specific age/sex related lifelong surveillance.
6.   Group activity
     (a)   Problem-related.
     (b)   Growth-related.
     (c)   Relationship-related.
     (d)   Work-related.
     (e)   Self-reliance promoting.
7.   Community development.
8.   Political action.
     (a)   Specific problems.
     (b)   Basic structures.

AN INDIVIDUALISTIC APPROACH

Every general practitioner wants to feel fulfilled in the work that he his doing, providing the best care he can for his patients, helping to signifi-cantly improve the quantity and quality of people's lives.

It is therefore with a great deal of dissatisfaction, even distress, that he frequently finds himself watching helplessly as his patients literally eat, drink, smoke and drive themselves into early graves or worse still, chronic disability. General practitioners find themselves involved mainly in 'crisis intervention', the frustrating business of trying to patch up broken bodies, minds and social relationships.

Realizing the limitations of secondary prevention (shutting stable doors after the horses have bolted), a general practitioner may decide upon primary prevention with his general practice population, believing that if only people could be shown what they were doing to themselves, before illness struck, they would change their ways and adopt healthier lifestyles. With this rather simplistic belief, he may embark on an ever-expanding search for effective tools for promoting health (McCamy and Presley, 1975).

How can the general practitioner organize his practice for preventive care?

Traditionally, in preventing disease, family doctors have been involved in:
1.   (a)   Patient education in routine consultations.
     (b)   Comprehensive diagnostic assessments.
2.   Immunization programmes.
3.   The 'annual medical' check-up.
4.   Influencing the environment – physically, socially and politically.

ROUTINE CONSULTING

Let us consider the routine doctor–patient consultation. If this is focussed on finding a diagnosis and technical management for the presenting problem, then ten minute appointments will probably be adequate.

The first step is simply to make time and use every opportunity to discuss with the patient the natural history of his or her disease, primary aetiological factors (cause–effect relationships) between health habits and symptoms and, most importantly, the very real limitations of medicine in reversing the process. Even a case of upper respiratory infection could provide an opportunity to enquire about smoking habits, diet, exercise, sleep, personal hygiene and so on.

A key question to ask in patient education is 'What is this illness saying to you about the way you are living?' In the crisis of ill-health, the patient is more open than usual to considering a change in his or her pattern of behaviour.

In the field of psychosocial health, useful questions include (Piggott, 1979):

'How happy do you feel?
"Mark on this five centimetre line how valuable you are to yourself (Y), to your spouse (S), to your friends (F)

NOT WORTH
ANYTHING ——————————————————————
MOST IMPORTANT
PERSON IN THE
WORLD

What do you feel about your relationships with your spouse?
With your work?
What about friends, do you have many? Any? How close are they? Are you able to discuss with them those things that matter most to you?'

Most patients appreciate this interest being shown in them, as intelligent and responsible people, and many are very receptive to the why, what and how of lifestyle change.

The smoker, the heavy drinker, the caffeine addict, or the sedentary businessman, for example, will often be more impressed by the relief from persistent bronchitis, peptic ulceration, tension headaches, irritability, lethargy or mild depression resulting from lifestyle modification, (avoiding chemicals, eating sensibly, making love, exercising regularly, learning to relax and so on), than from medication alone. Indeed, the more the general practitioner becomes involved in lifestyle correction as part of comprehensive medical care, the less he is tempted to use solely drug medication and surgery in the treatment of disease, while still applying the benefits of technology when essential.

In an unhurried consultation of about 20 minutes, there may be time for a comprehensive assessment, where the doctor can come to a common understanding with the patient of his/her state of physical, mental and social health, and its relationship to his/her way of life, work and interaction with the environment. This can lead the way to specific lifestyle planning, with the patient providing the values and decisions, while the doctor manages the process of practical decision making.

IMMUNIZATION PROGRAMMES

General practitioners have a key role to play in *monitoring* the immunization status of patients, promoting full cooperation of children and adults with public health authority immunization campaigns, as well as providing a service to individuals who request it, to ensure 'herd immunity' is achieved for communicable disease. Local protocols should be referred to for answers to the question '*Who* should be immunized *when*, for *what*?'

ANNUAL MEDICAL CHECK-UPS

Symptomatic patients are often well motivated, but what about the asymptomatic individual – the person, for example who presents for an 'annual medical'? These patients may be considered to fall into one of three categories:
1. Those who are already well motivated to do what they can to preserve their health.
2. Those who are interested only in finding out if they are healthy enough to continue their bad habits.
3. Those with mixed motives (the majority).

An all clear medical, excluding only the observable signs of existing disease, may serve only to confirm the majority of patients in their present self-destructive lifestyles.

The successful patient may even celebrate his good health with a visit to the pub, a meat pie and another carton of cigarettes on his way home. The more sophisticated the examination, the greater the reassurance. Patients often seem to interpret a normal electrocardiogram, for example, as evidence that the heart is normal, whereas, even with maximal exercise, false negatives may occur in 36 – 40% of men with anatomical evidence of coronary heart disease and clinical angina pectoris. Moreover, by the time such presymptomatic signs become evident, the disease process is usually well advanced and largely irreversible. Thus the annual medical check-up seems little better than a pat on the back.

Realizing these limitations of check-ups in primary prevention, the general practitioner may decide to look for *risk factors*, in either the lifestyle or measurable precursors, which would enable him to predict disease and hence prevent or delay its onset through control of such risk factors.

Assessment for health promotion can involve taking a family and personal history, making a physical examination and performing special tests (overlapping with presymptomatic detection and the early diagnosis and management of disease), but mainly looking for high risk problems for that individual.

Coronary risk profiles have provided one framework which general practitioners have taken up in the past. Using the American Heart Association's Coronary Risk Handbook, (American Heart Association, 1973) which is based on the Framingham Study, the probability of developing coronary heart disease in 6 years can be calculated from the patient's age, sex, smoking habits, blood pressure, serum cholesterol, electrocardiogram and glucose tolerance.

Additional risk factors can also be considered. These include history, personality type, relative weight, physical activity status and later, in at-risk patients, a stress test.

A positive stress test (i.e. a flat or negative ST depression of 1mm or greater) has been shown to have independent and additional predictive value. The risk ratio of a positive stress ECG over a negative stress ECG has been found to be as high as 21 times, on maximal tests, and 36 times, on submaximal tests. This is undoubtedly the most powerful predictor of coronary heart disease, provides a powerful incentive to control or eliminate other risk factors present, and especially to begin a well-planned and graduated walking programme. Those with a low aerobic power (maximal oxygen uptake) are likewise motivated to become more physically active.

In order to become proficient in exercise testing and prescription, nutrition, and behaviour modification techniques, a general practitioner will need to do some postgraduate courses. To fit in all of this, he may need to reduce his patient throughput below thirty consultations daily, take on an assistant and allocate certain times for performing risk profiles, for patient counselling and for study.

Although reasonably effective, coronary risk profiles have serious limitations:

1. They are too restricted, being confined to a single disease, and relevant mostly to males in the fourth and fifth decades of life.
2. The benefits, in terms of reduced risk of coronary heart disease through the control of risk factors, appear either marginal, at best, or unproven, at worst. Cigarette smoking, for example, is probably the most reversible of the risk factors. Yet, fewer than 10 pre-retirement coronary heart attacks would be prevented among 100 average 35-year old males who quit smoking. In other words, over 90% of them would have stopped in vain! The benefits (in terms of reduced incidence of coronary heart disease) from controlling elevated blood pressure and cholesterol levels, two other variables, are lower.

Such arguments, of course, ignore the total effects of cigarette smoking, a high fat diet and hypertension on other organs and diseases such as cancer of the lung, larynx, kidney and colon, hypertensive heart disease, cerebro-vascular accidents, renal failure and so on. What may be needed is a 'total risk profile', with specific personalized health education regarding known risks for the individual patient.

HEALTH RISK ASSESSMENT

The genius of prospective medicine is the 'Health Hazard Appraisal' (Robbins and Hall, 1970; Beeson and Phillips, 1977). This is a computed combination of all known risk factors for each of the top twelve or so causes of death, for each 5 year age group, for each sex, multiplied by the corresponding mean 10 year mortality risks for each cause of death and totalled, the total 10 year mortality risk being meaningfully expressed as a 'Health Appraisal Age', that is, the age of the 'average' person of the same sex and race, with that particular risk. The person is also given a 'Compliance Age', should he/she comply with the advice given to reduce excess risks.

The patient may also be shown how much 'younger' he/she can become with each change made. In a youth-oriented culture, the idea of 'growing younger' is very appealing and highly motivational for people over thirty, as has been demonstrated in several studies (La Dou, Sherwood and Hughes, 1975).

However, the general practitioner should be aware that Health Hazard Appraisal has significant difficulties for implementation:

1. Because it is based almost entirely on American data, it is necessary to substitute local mortality figures. This means eliminating some causes of death and adding others, (e.g. skin cancer in the tropics) for which precise risk factors may be difficult to determine and more difficult to combine.

2. The method used for combining individual risk factors is highly questionable, and possibly invalid statistically.

3. Without a computer, it is mathematically very cumbersome and time consuming. This can be partly overcome by redesigning the questionnaire in such a way that the patient does most of the calculations. This, of course, increases the likelihood of error. An alternative is to use a programmable calculator.

4. Sixty to ninety minute appointments are desirable. Thus the number of patients to be involved in Health Hazard Appraisal will be limited to perhaps five to ten each week.

5. It is disease-oriented. Some studies have actually shown that, whereas the 'fear of the consequences' of a disease (e.g. tuberculosis) is usually motivational, more often than not the 'fear of the disease itself' leads to denial and actually inhibits compliance with preventive measures.

Therefore, the emphasis is probably better shifted to a decidedly health-oriented approach.

Belloc and Breslow of the Human Population Laboratory, California State Department of Public Health, Berkeley, surveyed 6928 adults in Alamada County for 'health habits'. They found that just seven health practices were strongly correlated with health status which was a function of age (Belloc and Breslow, 1972).

Table 1   Morbidity risk ('Vitality Age') from Alamada Study

HEALTH HABITS: (score 'yes' answers)
1. □ I usually get 7 or 8 hours of sleep at night.
2. □ I eat breakfast almost every day.
3. □ I rarely or never eat in between my regular meals.
4. □ Females: I am not more than 10 per cent above my ideal weight.
       Males: I am between 95 and 120 per cent of my ideal weight.
5. □ I *often* engage in active sports, swimming, taking long walks, working in the garden or doing physical exercises.
6. □ I do not drink wine, beer or liquor . . . or . . .
       When I do, I usually have fewer than five drinks at one sitting.
7. □ I have never smoked cigarettes regularly.

TALLY: – –
VITALITY AGE: Find your score below and add (algebraically) to your actual age.

Age	0-2 Habits	3 Habits	4 Habits	5 Habits	6 Habits	7 Habits
20-24	+14.3	+ 7.4	+ 0.5	−1.1	−4.2	− 9.4
25-29	+15.6	+ 8.3	+ 1.8	−0.9	−4.5	−10.2
30-40	+16.9	+ 9.1	+ 3.0	−0.6	−4.7	−11.1
35-39	+18.2	+ 9.9	+ 4.2	−0.4	−5.0	−12.0
40-44	+19.4	+10.7	+ 5.4	−0.1	−5.2	−12.9
45-49	+20.7	+11.6	+ 6.7	+0.1	−5.5	−13.8
50-54	+22.0	+12.4	+ 7.9	+0.3	−5.7	−14.7
55-59	+23.3	+13.2	+ 9.1	+0.6	−6.0	−15.5
60-64	+24.5	+14.0	+10.4	+0.8	−6.2	−16.4
65-69	+25.8	+14.8	+11.6	+1.1	−6.5	−17.3
70-74	+27.1	+15.7	+12.8	+1.3	−6.8	−18.2

From the health habit questionnaire above, plus the scoring system and evaluation tables derived from the findings of the Alameda study, an individual can very simply determine his morbidity risk or 'vitality age'.

Thus a 60-year old male who did not smoke, usually drank less than five alcoholic drinks per sitting, regularly ate breakfast, seldom or never ate between meals, was not overweight, was often physically active, and who usually had 7 or 8 hours sleep at night, had the same physical health status score as a 30-year old male with fewer than three of these habits.

Rational motivation to improve one's vitality age by improving one's health habits assumes a causal relationship. Although this was not proven by the study, a 9½ year follow-up study is suggestive.

MOTIVATION

The key reason for using such health evaluations is to motivate the patient to change his/her lifestyle. A further useful step is to acquire a number of motivational and educational aids. These may include audiotape or cassette–slide audiovisuals (on diet, exercise, obesity and weight control, smoking, tension, rest, relaxation and general health principles), and literature relating to common risk factors (e.g. smoking, hyperlipidaemia, hypertension and so on, their significance and methods of control), and common health problems (e.g. acne, arthritis, diverticulitis, headaches, heartburn, insomnia, peptic ulcer and so on, with an emphasis upon self-care and lifestyle modification). These will supplement individual health counselling. Patients seem to find the advice of a doctor who has carried out a comprehensive assessment as very motivational. An abnormal stress electrocardiogram has also been found to be highly motivating to a patient to change his lifestyle.

How can the general practitioner assess whether his patient will be motivated to live in a health-promoting manner? One introductory approach to this question is provided by 'The Health Script', developed from Transactional Analysis theory:

The HEALTH SCRIPT questionnaire (Marx, Barnes, Somers and Garrity, 1978)

1. If you continue the way you are going, where will you be in 5 years with regard to your health?
2. How often in the past have you been sick?
3. When you were sick, how did your parents react to you?
4. During the next year do you think you will get sick or depressed?
5. How often do you remember your mother or dad getting sick?
6. When your dad got sick, how did mother react? When your mother got sick, how did dad react?
7. How did your parents react to a family crisis? That is, what did they do when things got tough?
8. What do you remember as the nicest thing your mother or dad ever said to you or did for you when you were sick?
9. What do you remember as the worst thing your mother or dad ever said to you or did to you when you were sick?
10. What do you recall as the main advice regarding how to stay healthy that you got from your parents?
11. What is the advice YOU would give people about how to stay physically and mentally healthy?
12. What do you predict will be the probable cause of your death?
13. At what age do you predict you will die?

(The patient should be instructed to answer each of these questions 'straight off the top of his head', within four seconds, to enable access to the 'automatic, programmed Parent/Child' data. These questions are not meant to be analysed rationally by the patient.)

A general practitioner who detects that his patient has been 'programmed' by his parents for a sick-role or self-destruction, should prepare the patient for psychological counselling, and not waste his time further on rational persuasion.

SPECIFIC AGE/SEX RELATED LIFELONG SURVEILLANCE

What of the future? For several years, the Royal Australian College of General Practitioners' Preventive and Community Medicine Committee has been studying lifetime health surveillance, (*Australian Family Physician*, 1979) focusing attention on the question: 'What are the major preventable conditions for each sex and age group – from the antenatal period until death?' The College is in the process of preparing its own list of target conditions with recommended interventions. The Committee considers that all general practitioners can carry out these surveillance measures 'in passing', when the patient is attending anyway for unrelated symptoms. This will achieve an annual population coverage close to 70%, and over 90% in a five year period, in advanced Western countries, compared with the highly-motivated 15% who attend for specific 'check-ups'. It has become the pattern for 'dependent groups' such as children and the elderly to have a specific timetable recommended for them. This proposal is to extend health promotion to all age groups.

The development of an age–sex register for the practice population is a useful tool if comprehensive lifetime health surveillance and periodic health examinations are to be offered to the community, to enable the doctor to know when to offer the service or to request particular patients to attend.

To enable doctors in each country to develop their own lists, detailed recommendations regarding the Periodic Health Examination can be obtained from a variety of sources, some of which are mentioned below.

Hilleboe, H.E. 'Modern Concepts of Prevention in Community Health' *Am. J. Public Hlth.* May 1971 has suggested a preliminary check-list of possible preventive actions.

Breslow, L. and Somers, A. In 'The Lifetime Health Monitoring Programme. A Practical Approach to Preventive Medicine' *N. Engl. J. Med.*, March 17, 1977 use clinical and epidemiological criteria to identify specific health goals and professional services appropriate for ten different age groups.

The Report of the Canadian Task Force on the Periodic Health Examination, *Canadian Medical Association Journal, Vol.*, 121, 1979 provides a most comprehensive set of recommendations and rationale. Some examples of suggested 'Health Protection Packages' are given below in Table 64MR and Table 64M, and quoted in the relevant age-related sections. 'Healthy People' The Surgeon General's 1978 Report on Health Promotion and Disease Prevention in the United States of America, was followed by specific 'Objectives for the Nation' for promoting health and preventing disease. Some of these are quoted in the next section. Readers are referred to these publications for details, obtainable from the US Department of Health and Human Services.

HEALTH PROTECTION PACKAGE (64M)

Number	Target condition	Manoeuvres	Best current estimate of optimal frequency	Remarks (if any)
MEN Age 45–64 years As for age 16–44 years Plus:				
64M1	Cancer of the colon and rectum (B)	Testing of occult blood in stools	Not more frequently than annually	High research priority, determine the sensitivity specificity, accept side, effects and appropriate frequency for detection tests
64M2	Retirement distress (C)	Final examination before retirement as part of a series of periodic health examinations	Once	

Considerable discussion on the efficacy of routine testing of apparently healthy adults has resulted so far in no definite lead being given by responsible authorities. Some advocate expensive screening, others doubt effectiveness in any programme. Certainly there are some patients – 'the worried well', for example – who appear to receive too much attention; others progress through life unaware of dangerous situations, such as increasing hypertension. Sometimes these are brought to notice by chance during a minor episode of illness (Cormack, Marinker and Morrell, 1976).

The frequency of assessment below is offered as a guide for a balanced programme of care, and to provoke discussion relevant to your own situation. The editors invite comments and suggestions.

Young adults (aged 15–40):   attendance every 5 years
Middle age (40–60):   attendance every 2 years
Older adults (over 60):   annual attendance

The RACGP Health Record System (RACGP, 1976), and 'A Manual for General Practice' by Selwyn Carson (Carson, 1979) in its recent Australian, New Zealand and United Kingdom editions, provide readily

HEALTH PROTECTION PACKAGE (64MR)

Number	Target condition	Manoeuvre	Best current estimate of optimal frequency	Remarks if (any)
MEN Age 16-44 years **High-risk groups**				
64MR1	Immunizable conditions related to international travel (A)	Immunization	See corresponding summary for specific indications in the complementary report	
64MR2	Tuberculosis	Tuberculin sensitivity testing, BCG immunization and chemoprophylaxis as necessary	On the basis of clinical judgement	In people exposed to disease through their work, in contact with infected people, or living in communities with a high infection rate.
64MR3	Gonorrhea	Smears of urethra, culture of urethral secretions and of first-voided urine	At appropriate intervals on the basis of clinical judgement	Persons in the military, work camps and prisons; homosexuals
64MR4	Syphilis	Serological testing	At appropriate intervals on the basis of clinical judgement	Persons in the military, work camps and prisons; homosexuals
64MR5	Malnutrition	History, measurement of height and weight	At appropriate intervals on the basis of clinical judgement	Indians; Inuits; people in low socioeconomic conditions; food faddists
64MR6	Cancer of the skin	Inspection, counselling	At appropriate intervals on the basis of clinical judgement	People who work outdoors who are in contact with polycyclic aromatic hydrocarbons

available recommendations regarding frequency of examination, and proforma questionnaires.

CONSULTATION PLAN

Routine care at any age has specific areas of interest related to that age, in terms of early detection of conditions especially liable to occur, or initially detectable in that particular age group. Specifically requested 'check-up' well patient examinations enable full advantage to be taken of the opportunity for both early pre-symptom detection of disease and also health promotion, with specific reference to both examination procedures and counselling requirements according to age and sex.

GENERAL RECOMMENDATIONS

1. *Consideration of the health goals of that particular age group*

2. *History*

In addition to traditional medical data, lifestyle and environmental information is of great importance. Smoking and alcohol, diet, including fast foods and fat intake, 'time budgeting', physical activity patterns, both at work and recreation, and personality type (A or B), are extremely important in determining predisposition to disease, as well as providing an excellent basis for health promotion.

3. *Physical examination including any special tests*

Weight, blood pressure and urine testing, as well as particular attention to any elucidated symptoms.

4. *Counselling session*

(a)   Explaining what information has been obtained.
(b)   Providing health education as generally applicable to the age group
        (e.g. breast or testicle self-examination).
(c)   Followed by individual counselling and treatment, if required.

The next section details specific recommendations for specific age groups, from antenatal care through to the elderly.

HEALTHY INFANTS

Consider these general strategies:

Education for parenthood

People who are well informed about the care required by infants can better plan and prepare for parenthood. Prospective parents can seek education-for-parenthood classes from doctors, hospitals, and community organizations. Schools can offer preparation for parenthood to children and teenagers.

Prenatal care

Good prenatal care is essential for a healthy pregnancy. Medical care, dietary assistance and counselling are important for all expectant mothers.

Mothers with social and economic barriers to such care can be identified by family doctors for special follow-up.

Prenatal nutrition

Pregnant women have extra needs for iron, protein, calcium, and calories and may need to be provided with dietary suggestions and/or supplements.

Condition	Manoeuvre
Postnatal asphyxia	Detection during pregnancy of causative factors suggesting high risk (see list). Fetal monitoring during labour
Hemorrhagic disease of the newborn	Vitamin K_1, 1 mg after birth
Congenital syphilis	Serologic testing
Ophthalmia neonatorum (gonococcal)	Instillation of 1% silver nitrate solution into each eye
Neonatal hypothyroidism	Thyroxine testing with filter paper in all neonates; ancillary spot testing for thyroid stimulating hormone if necessary
Phenylketonuria	For detection, microbiologic inhibition (Guthrie) and fluorometric tests; may need repeating and supplementing with paper chromatography
Congenital dislocation of hip	Clinical examination (flexion, abduction and Ortolani manoeuvre); confirmation by X-ray
Neural tube defect	Maternal serum alphafetoprotein testing; with elevated values, supplement with ultrasound and amniocentesis
Cystic fibrosis	Detection: iontophoresis sweat test on at least two occasions, and observation for clinical signs
Duchenne muscular dystrophy (DMD)	Serum creatine phosphokinase determination
Interventricular septal defect (VSD)	History taking and clinical examination; chest X-ray and cardiac catheterization for confirmation
Tay-Sachs disease	Measurement of resistance of serum hexosaminidase to heat inactivation; amniocentesis as confirmatory test
Down's syndrome	Elicit information on patient's history; if positive, amniocentesis only if parents are prepared to accept abortion when it is indicated
Consequences in children of parents with alcoholism	Counselling to reduce alcohol intake; contraception for alcoholic, sexually active women; abortion may be considered for pregnant women at high risk
Low birth weight	Ensure adequacy of protein and energy intake; advise mother to abstain from or reduce smoking
Congenital herpes simplex	Caesarian section may be advisable for mothers with active genital herpes infection

Prenatal maternal habits

To reduce the potential for adverse effects on the developing fetus, women should avoid tobacco and alcohol during pregnancy. Counselling and appropriate services can help expectant mothers who wish to avoid these risks. Similarly, doctors should avoid prescribing medications and exposure to radiation by pregnant women, unless warranted by special circumstances.

Amniocentesis

A test (amniocentesis) sampling the intrauterine fluid at about the 16th week of pregnancy can determine whether certain serious birth defects exist in the fetus. Expectant mothers at higher risk include those who: are 35 and over; have a history of multiple spontaneous abortions; or have a family history of Down's syndrome, neural tube defects or inherited disorders. Detection of an abnormality may require a personal decision about an abortion.

Consider these specific conditions in neonates.

Age group 0-4

Suggested consultation at six weeks, four, six, nine and eighteen months two, three and four years.

Health goals

1. To establish immunity against specified infectious diseases.
2. To detect and prevent certain other diseases and problems before irreparable damage occurs.
3. To facilitate growth and development to the infant's optimal potential. Every GP should take every opportunity of appreciating the capabilities of normal infants and children. Thus, at any consultation, he can look for and recognize defects outside the range of normal.
4. To provide a basis for lifelong emotional stability; especially through a loving relationship within the family.

Consider these general strategies:

Social services

Some families require special support services to enhance the healthy growth and development of their children. Such services include high quality day care, improved foster care and adoption programme, as well as services to assist families in which a parent may suffer from chronic disabling disease, mental illness, alcoholism, or drug abuse.

Preventive counselling of the mother may follow the guidelines from Kevin Cullen on 'Prevention of Behaviour Problems in Preschool Children' (Cullen, 1975). Prevention of accidents in the home should be considered.

Condition	Manoeuvre
Immunizable infectious diseases:	
Diphtheria	Immunization of persons in good health
Measles	Immunization of persons in good health
Mumps	Immunization of persons in good health
Pertussis	Immunization of persons in good health
Poliomyelitis	Immunization of persons in good health
Rubella	Immunization of children and/or girls and women at risk
Tetanus	Immunization of persons in good health
Influenza	Immunization
Pneumococcal meningitis	Immunization
Meningococcal meningitis	Immunization

*Routine preventive care in the first 15 years of life**

Age	Doctor	Practice staff	Present schedule of childhood immunization
Birth	X		
2 weeks	X	X	
6 weeks	X	X	
4 months		X	Trivac. Polio
6 months		X	Trivac. Polio
9 months	X	X	
1 year	X	X	Measles/Mumps
18 months		X	Dip-Tet. Polio
3 years		X	
5 years	X	X	Dip-Tet.
7 years		X	
10 years	X ·	X	Rubella (girls)
15 years	X	X	Tetanus/Rubella (girls)

*This table is recommended by Australian health authorities. Variations may occur in other countries. Readers should seek the advice of the health authorities in their own country.

Breast feeding

Breast milk is the most complete form of infant nutrition and is recommended for full-term newborn babies, unless there are specific problems or breast feeding is unsuccessful. If a nursing mother is healthy and well nourished, fluoride and possibly Vitamin D may be the only supplements needed by the baby. After about four months iron also may have to be added. Solid foods should not be introduced hastily into a baby's diet – rather they should be phased in gradually.

Immunization

Childhood diseases that can be prevented by vaccinations continue to be a threat to infant health. Babies should be immunized for diphtheria, pertussis, tetanus, and polio at ages two months, four months, and six months (polio immunization is optional at six months). They should also receive the recommended childhood immunizations thereafter (see NH & MRC list).

HEALTHY CHILDREN

Consider these general strategies:

Early childhood development

A stimulating and healthy environment during the early part of life can enhance a child's growth and development. Programmes such as the Kindergartens and Early Childhood Development Programme, which provide comprehensive services for children, including day care, health care, nutrition, education and counselling, have produced important gains in child development, particularly for families with low incomes.

Special support services

Special sources of support should be available through community agencies and family doctors to assist children and families under particular stress.

Injury reduction

Accidents are the single greatest threat to children's health. People can reduce children's risk of injury and death by:
  *having the child secured in an approved child carrier, safety harness or seat belt when travelling in an automobile;
  *storing toxic agents out of reach, away from food, and in special containers with fastened safety caps;

*ensuring against access to knives and guns;
*carefully supervising young children at play, particularly when they are near water or streets;
*instructing the child what to do in situations of special risk (e.g. stoves, matches, electrical sockets, traffic).

Healthy habits

Preparing young children for peer group pressures with regard to smoking, alcohol use, and sexual activity can enhance their ability to deal with those pressures later. Parents, schools, and family doctors are all important to the provision of comprehensive health education which can help children to acquire skills to cope with problems they will confront as teenagers.

Nutrition and exercise

Acquiring healthy eating and exercise habits in childhood may have lifelong benefits. An appropriate balance of food intake and physical activity promotes normal weight. Excessive intake of salt, sugar, and fats should be avoided. Parents and schools can emphasize these points through instruction, meal planning, and physical education programmes emphasizing lifelong exercise activities. Nutrition supplements can be provided to children in high risk families.

Fluoridation

The most effective and efficient way to prevent tooth decay is through fluoridation of community water supplies. If the water supply is not fluoridated, alternative fluoride sources can be provided through school-based fluoride mouth rinse or tablet programmes, fluoride rinsing services from dentists, and fluoride tablets for home use.

Dental care

Children should be taught proper tooth brushing and flossing techniques at early ages, and should begin regular visits to a dentist by age three. Sweets in the diet should be limited to prevent tooth decay.

Annual screening

Age 1–4 annual screening in addition to episodal attendance. Purpose-screening for congenital or acquired abnormalities. Early screening for specific learning disabilities. Counselling mother on preschool child behaviour patterns for prevention of behaviour problems. Early referral for problems of speech, hearing or sight. Prevention of accidents in the home is again worth discussing with mother.

Age Group 1-4

10 Year Risks of Death: Accidents – 175; Cancer – 45;
(per 100 000)   All other diseases – 160

Paediatric care

Some childhood problems can be prevented or ameliorated through the
provision of certain medical services. Examples of such services include:
identification and treatment of vision and hearing problems; assessment of
developmental skills important to learning; immunizations and early diagnosis and treatment of childhood infections.

Consider these specific conditions in preschool children

Condition	Manoeuvre
Obesity in childhood	Accurate serial measurements of height and weight
Problems of physical growth (hormonal)	Serial measurements of height and weight and other anthropometric measurements
Parenting problems, including child abuse and neglect	Appropriate history taking, counselling and assessment of parent–child interaction
Hyperactivity and learning disability	Assess parent–child interaction: preschool educational screening
Strabismus	Simple inspection and cover–uncover test
Haemolytic streptococcal infection resulting in acute glomerulonephritis or acute rheumatic fever	Elicit history of exposure to beta-haemolytic streptococcal infection; throat culture
Urinary tract infection	Urinalysis
Toxoplasmosis	Elicit information on exposure; serologic testing for *Toxoplasma gondii* and counselling on hygiene for high-risk group

Age group 5-9

10 Year Risks of Death: Accidents – 135; Cancer – 45;
(per 100 000)   All other diseases – 110

Providing screening has been adequate to age five, a five year interval is
justifiable. However, if abnormalities have been detected, either physical
or behavioural, annual checks may continue to be beneficial to both
mother and child. Mothers should be encouraged to return should
behavioural problems arise during the primary school years. The main
dangers to this group are still accidents, particularly on the roads and in
the water. The importance of diet in promoting resistance to disease and in
the prevention of obesity should be stressed.

Consider these specific conditions in primary school children:

Condition	Manoeuvre
Dental	Visual and tactile examination, and X-rays if appropriate. Fluoride application for residents of areas without fluoridated water supply. Water fluoridation
Orthodontic conditions	Oral examination and encouragement of daily oral hygiene
Periodontal disease	Visual and tactile examination and encouragement of daily oral hygiene

Age group 10–14

10 Year Risks of Death:
(per 100 000)

Accidents – 340; Suicide – 45;
Cancer – 45;
All other diseases – 170

One check during this period may be sufficient for the normal child. Parents may wish for advice on pubertal changes, and on changing parent child relationships.

HEALTHY ADOLESCENTS AND YOUNG ADULTS

Consider these general strategies:

Roadway safety

Automobile accidents are the leading cause of death among young people. A substantial number of injuries and deaths could be avoided through careful, defensive driving habits. Especially important are: avoiding driving after drinking (or riding with a driver who has been drinking) or use of mood-altering drugs; obeying traffic laws; and using seat belts or, for motorcyclists, helmets. These efforts can be reinforced by Federal, State and local measures to set and enforce safety regulations and lower speed limits, and to improve roadway and vehicular design.

Smoking, alcohol, and drug use

Experimental behaviour by young people can lead to dependence or misuse of certain substances. Collective measures can be taken by parents, teachers, doctors, and community organizations to provide adolescents and young adults with information and skills necessary to help them avoid cigarette smoking or harmful use of alcohol or drugs.

Nutrition and exercise

Changes in values and social pressures may encourage adolescents to eat snack foods that do not contain adequate supplies of essential nutrients. Yet, good eating habits and regular, vigorous exercise are important to still growing adolescents. During their growth spurt, teenagers need more calories, and particularly more protein, calcium and iron.

Family planning

Unwanted pregnancy is a distressing problem for adolescent and young adult women in this country. Families, schools, doctors, and social organizations can ensure that information about birth control measures is provided to young people of both sexes, and that family planning services are easily accessible to those who are sexually active. Services (including continued schooling) can also be made available in the community for young women who become pregnant and are in need of care and advice.

Sexually transmissible diseases

Sexually transmissible diseases that affect large numbers of young people are preventable. Families, schools, doctors and social organizations can help provide information, confidential counselling, and treatment to prevent the transmission of venereal diseases. Periodic screening for disease which may not be symptomatic can be obtained from family doctors and community clinics, and encouraged for sexually active young people. Clinic personnel, sex educators, and family planning services counsellors can stress the value of condoms in reducing the spread of disease and can emphasize the importance of informing partners immediately if disease is discovered.

Immunization

Young people should receive booster immunization for diphtheria and tetanus at age 15.

Mental health

Young people frequently experience periods of frustration, uncertainty, and confusion, and should be encouraged to talk over problems. Alert and sensitive friends, family members, clergy, or counsellors at work can be helpful during periods of stress, anxiety, depression or uncertainty. 'Hotlines' may also be helpful. Mental health professionals may be needed if conditions persist.

Firearms

Handguns are involved in a substantial number of homicides, suicides and accidental deaths in this country. Actions at the individual, community, and governmental levels can provide measures to reduce the availability of handguns.

Age group 15–19

10 Year Risks of Death: Accidents – 630; Suicide – 120;
(per 100 000)   All other diseases – 230

In the absence of signs and symptoms, screening for disease is unlikely to be productive.

Health goals

1. Preventive medicine should deal with the main hazards of the age – drugs, alcohol and driving.
2. Opportunity should be given for any sexual problems or relationship difficulties to be discussed.
3. Problems of employment, future goals and self-image may need to be talked out.

Consider these specific conditions in late teenagers:

Condition	Manoeuvre
Parasitic diseases, excluding toxoplasmosis	No specific manoeuvre Hygiene
Gonorrhea	Smears of cervix, vagina, rectum and urethra for Gram stain and culture of secretions. Look at first-voided urine
Syphilis	Various blood tests
Chlamydial genital infection	Blood tests, cultures and smears
Herpes virus type 2 and cytomegalovirus infection	Blood tests, cultures and microscopy
Unwanted teenage pregnancy	Counselling on contraceptive use and follow-up; abortion
Scoliosis	Physical inspection in schools by nurses or by family doctor

Checklist

Infectious diseases
Glandular fever, infectious hepatitis.
Rubella immunization for teenage girls – have they slipped through the net at school?
Acne.

Nutritional
Care of teeth.
Anorexia nervosa or feeding/weight problems.
Inadequate diet from diversion of income to leisure activities.
Obesity.
Leisure activities
Sporting injuries.
Loud music.
Driving problems: drink, motorcycles, drug effects.
Smoking.
Alcoholism.
Drug misuse, willfully or in ignorance.
Occupational
Specific occupational injuries – e.g. back strain, eye injuries – and prophylaxis.
Problems of unemployment.
Changing jobs.
Further education.
Sexual
Contraception.
Sexually transmitted disease.
Sexual inadequacy.
Sexual orientation problems – "Am I a homosexual?"
Dysmenorrhoea.
Unwanted pregnancy.
Behaviour and mental health
Realistic view of self, intelligence and capabilities.
Relationships with family, and sexual partners and friends.
Loneliness, depression.
Suicide, parasuicide, self-injury.
Drug abuse.

Age group 20-24

10 Year Risks of Death: Accidents – 530; Suicide – 160;
(per 100 000)   Cancer – 70;
                                 All other diseases – 310

Examine once during this time, preferably before employment, university entrance, or marriage.

Health goals

Transition from adolescence to maturity with maximum physical, mental and emotional resources, and full capacity for healthy marriage, parenthood and social relationships.

Standards for health maintenance to be thought about at this stage, before patterns become fixed. Weight, diet, exercise and relaxation, interests and hobbies, anything leading to a balanced and satisfying lifestyle. In the future one will not have to wait till retirement to consider the best use of leisure time. Marriage problems may arise in this age group and early counselling may prevent later disruption. Pregnancy allows for many counselling opportunities with women.

Professional services

Full standard physical examination including urine test, blood pressure, obesity assessment, height/weight relationship (preferably percentage body fat) and eye tests (including colour blindness), and musculoskeletal capacity including flexibility. Dental examination by dentist. Special tests – blood for VD tests and cholesterol level. Further tests according to individual need. Cervical smear. All adults should be advised to maintain tetanus immunity.

Counselling on diet, exercise, work, occupational hazards, sex, alcohol, drugs, smoking, driving and interpersonal relationships.

HEALTHY ADULTS

Consider these general strategies: quoted from the 'Healthy People' summary of measures for better health.

Smoking

Cigarette smoking is the principal preventable cause of chronic disease and death in this country. Public education efforts at the Federal, State and local levels, as well as by family doctors, can provide information about the health hazards of smoking and suggestions on how to stop. Those who cannot quit on their own may benefit from one of the organized smoking cessation clinics. Those who are unable or unwilling to stop ought to smoke brands low in tar and nicotine, to inhale less, to smoke their cigarettes only halfway, and to reduce gradually the number of cigarettes smoked. Doctors' instructions to stop smoking definitely help.

Alcohol

Misuse of alcohol leads to accidental injury, family disruption, and chronic disease for millions of people. It is important that people realize the dangers – particularly for pregnant women – when alcohol is used excessively. Individuals (or their families) with alcohol-related problems may find effective assistance from health professionals the clergy, community groups such as Alcoholics Anonymous, or programmes run by various businesses to assist employees with drinking problems.

Nutrition

Good nutrition is an essential component of good health. People should adopt prudent dietary habits, consuming:

*only sufficient calories to meet body needs (fewer calories if the person is overweight);

*less saturated fat and cholesterol;

*less salt;

*less sugar;

*relatively more complex carbohydrates, such as whole grains, cereals, fruit and vegetables;

*relatively more fish, poultry, legumes (e.g. péas, beans, peanuts), and less red meat.

Employers, food advertisers, grocery stores, and health and social service agencies can add to the promotion of healthy nutritional habits by providing the information and access to foods necessary to a good diet.

Exercise

Regular exercise can bring physical and psychological benefits. Adults should be encouraged to exercise vigorously – if possible, at least three times a week for about 15 – 30 minutes each time. However, caution should be taken to initiate activity gradually, and anyone over 40, or with a health problem of any kind, should consult a doctor before beginning a vigorous exercise programme. The importance of regular and sustained exercise for adults should be stressed in public information programmes and by doctors. Communities and employers can encourage fitness related programmes, including, where practical, the provision of facilities or pathways to make bicycling, running, and other exercise safer and more convenient.

Environmental health

Toxic agents in our environment can present health hazards which may not be detected for years. Private and public actions at all levels are important to protect against possible environmental hazards. Individuals can support the monitoring of industrial and agricultural production processes to reduce exposure to potentially toxic agents.

Worksite health and safety

The occupational setting is important both as a source of potential health hazards and a site for health promotion activities. Health programmes at the worksite can provide information and protection related to all potential workplace hazards for employees, including stress, as well as offer activities and services to promote healthier lifestyles. People should both encourage these programmes and take advantage of them. Lower Workers Compensation insurance premiums are one result.

Hypertension

High blood pressure affects millions of people and is a major contributor to heart disease and stroke. Adults should have a screening examination for high blood pressure at least every five years, and every two to three years if over age 40. If hypertension is discovered, and medication prescribed, it is important that people follow their therapeutic regimens carefully. Doctors need to optimize their skills and practice procedures to ensure patient adherence.

Pap smear

The Pap smear is an important tool to detect cervical cancer at early stages. Women should have three Pap smears taken one year apart beginning at age 20, or at the beginning of sexual activity. Thereafter, a Pap smear should be taken every three years. Screening frequency should be increased if any abnormalities are found, or if a woman is taking oral contraceptives or oestrogen therapy.

Breast examination

Self-examination is the most effective way to detect breast cancer at an early treatable stage. Women should examine their own breasts monthly after the menstrual period, for early signs of cancer (lumps, abnormal discharge, irregular size). Postmenopausal women should select a specific day of the month for such self-examination. Family doctors and public health education programmes can provide information and instruction on breast self-examination, and increase their efforts to disseminate this important information. Periodic screening by mammography is not needed until after age 50, except for women who have already had cancer in one breast, and after 40 for women with a family history of breast cancer.

Cancer signs

Some cancers present signs at early stages in which the chances for successful treatment are greater. People should watch for early signs of cancer and consult a doctor if any are noticed. In addition to the signs for breast cancer noted above, other cancer signs include: changes in bowel or bladder habits; a sore that does not heal; unusual bleeding or discharge; difficulty swallowing; change in a wart or mole, or a nagging cough or hoarseness.

Mental health

Many people suffer from various forms of emotional disorders or mental illness. It is quite common for people to become, at one time or another, uncommonly anxious, depressed, or have difficulty coping with a life event. Professional assistance may be helpful if particular difficulty is encountered and may be available from family doctors, employers, local media, community organizations, hospitals, telephone 'hotlines' and other 'outreach' organizations.

Dental care

People frequently lose their teeth prematurely because of poor dental and gum care. Adults should take care of their teeth with daily brushing and flossing and an annual dental examination.

Specific procedures

The plan should be to record basic data at 5 year intervals (that is ten times between 20 and 64 years).

Basic data set
Height
Weight
Blood pressure
Urine – albumin/glucose
Vision
Hearing
Blood – haemoglobin/lipids

Females
Cervical smear
Breasts
Males
Testes
Prostate
Personal data: opportunity for your
patient to report
Health – symptoms?
Habits – smoking?
Habits – alcohol?
Habits – exercise?
Habits – diet?
Work – nature?
Marriage – sex?
Home – ?
Family – children?
Parents – health and dependence?

Check-list

Programme has to be designed.

Practice staff have to be allocated shared work (who does what?).

Patients have to be informed and invited to participate.

Recording system has to be devised.

Arrangements for the data recording to be made either at regular consultations or at special session.

Abnormalities must be followed up.

Re-examination every five years to be organized.

Young middle-age 25-39 years

Examine every 5 years.

Health goals

Maximization of total potential, prolongation of the period of maximum

Consider these specific conditions in young middle age:

Condition	Manoeuvre
Immunizable conditions related to international travel (smallpox, cholera, yellow fever, typhus, plague, typhoid and hepatitis)	Immunization (note contraindications); gammaglobulin against hepatitis
Tuberculosis	BCG immunization and chemoprophylaxis
Malnutrition	History taking, height and weight measurement and other anthropometric measurements and determination of serum protein concentration for high risk groups
Family dysfuncion and marital and sexual problems	History taking and counselling
Psychiatric disorders (affective disorders and suicide)	No predictive manoeuvre is available
Smoking	History taking and counselling
Alcohol consumption	History taking and counselling
Refractive defects	Visual acuity testing
Hearing defects	History taking and clinical examination
Recurrent spontaneous abortion	Investigation to detect possible cause of problem
Bacteriuria in pregnancy	Microbiological examination of urine
Preterm labour	Elicit previous history; culture of cervix; pharmacologic treatment; delivery in specialized centre
Blood group incompatibility in pregnancy	Blood group and antibody tests

energy. Prevention of chronic disease by health promotion and early detection and treatment.

Counselling

Diet, exercise, smoking, alcohol, emotional aspects of health-related lifestyle.

Self-examination

Breasts, skin, testes, neck and mouth.

Professional services

1. Full standard examination.
2. Special tests:
   Electrocardiogram.
   Take blood (fasting) for cholesterol
   and triglyceride examination.
3. Advise dental examination.
4. Other tests if indicated.

Cervical smears should be performed every 3 years.

Age group 25–29

10 Year Risks of Death: Accident – 370; Suicide – 160;
(per 100 000)   Cancer – 130; Vascular disease – 80;
                                    All other diseases – 3000

Consider these general issues:
The problems discussed remain as in the previous five years, but it is likely that in this group family problems predominate. Problems of young children, husband–wife problems, working wives and stay-home wives. Early drinking problems may show up, and smoking habits may be abandoned before physical damage is done. Individual responsibility for health may be accepted at this stage.

Age group 30–39

10 Year Risks of Death: Accidents – 630; Suicide – 300;
(per 100 000)   Heart diseases – 490; Cancer 560

Consider these general issues:
Many adults will be at the busiest stage of their careers, and may be unwilling to attend for screening unless their employment necessitates it, or special procedures, such as Pap smear, serve as reminders. Counselling

will be on health maintenance and disease prevention. Obesity may become a problem especially if pressure of work precludes the taking of regular physical exercise.

Serum cholesterol levels are worth monitoring from here on, and health hazards should be minimised if possible. Stress may lead to symptoms pointing the way to organised illness such as peptic ulcer. Early detection of this may lead to counter measures such as relaxation, yoga and recreation. Parents may have problems with adolescent or teenage children which they wish to discuss.

Consider these specific conditions in young middle age:

Condition	Manoeuvre
Diabetes mellitus in the non-pregnant adult	Urine testing for glucose: fasting, after blood glucose test, and after meal
Hyperthyroidism	Measurement of serum thyroxine and triiodo-thyronine concentrations and thyroid binding globulin saturation index
Hyperlipidaemia	Taking family history in young males and determining serum cholesterol and triglyceride concentrations
Hypertension	Blood pressure measurement; evaluation and treatment as appropriate
Thalassaemia	History taking, laboratory screening and counselling
Iron deficiency anaemia	Determination of blood haemoglobin concentration
Chronic bronchitis	Encourage abstinence from smoking
Alpha-1-antitrypsin deficiency	Encourage abstinence from smoking
Ankylosing spondylitis	Detection of individuals with HLA-B27 antigen
Rheumatoid arthritis	Unclear
Peptic ulcer	Elicit history
Cholelithiasis	For primary prevention, duodenal drainage of bile (limited use); for secondary prevention, oral cholecystography ± duodenal drainage
Cancer of the skin	Inspection; counselling
Cancer of the colon and rectum	Occult blood in stools, rectal examination

OLDER MIDDLE-AGE 40–59 YEARS

Full examination every 5 years with basic screening annually; and that for cervical, breast, and intestinal cancer every 2 years.

Health goals

Prolongation of physical capacity and mental and social activity, including adjustment to the menopause. Early detection of any chronic major disease.

Counselling

Self-monitoring reinforced by regular annual visits.

Professional services

1. Full standard examination.
2. Particular attention to cardiovascular disease, notably, coronary disease; and its production by diet, inactivity, stress, and smoking.
3. Careful screening for neoplastic disease.
4. Other tests if indicated.

Age group 40–49

10 Year Risks of Death: Heart disease – 2250; Cancer – 1850;
(per 100 000)   Accidents – 620; Suicide – 380

Consider these general issues:
During this period parents face the fact that they are ageing, their children have moved out and are entering their own reproductive cycle. The wife is facing menopausal problems, both may feel that they have grown apart, and need to establish a new relationship. Screening for cancer and heart disease become important at this age, and the physical component of the interview may expand from this time on.

Age group 50–59

10 Year Risks of Death: Heart disease – 7350; Cancer – 5000;
(per 100 000)   Accidents – 700

Consider these general issues:
Men may be at the peak of their career, but should be encouraged to think about how they will handle retirement. Careful screening for cardio-respiratory problems and cancer must be undertaken, and ECG, X-ray and spirometry may be justifiable screening procedures.

HEALTHY OLDER ADULTS

Consider these general strategies:

Work and social activity

Employment and/or volunteer opportunities are important for older people accustomed to working. Maintaining an active social life is also

Proposed check-list for health supervision of 40–60-year olds

Target condition	Strongly recommended procedure
Alcoholism	History and counselling
Smoking	History and counselling
Motor vehicle accident	History and counselling
Marital/family/sexual problems	History and counselling
Hearing loss	History and counselling
Hypertension	Measure B.P. and urine test
Carcinoma of cervix	Cervical smear
Dental caries	Dental examination and counselling
Diabetes	Fasting blood sugar and urine test

Target condition	Recommended procedure
Obesity/malnutrition	History and measure weight and counselling
Carcinoma of uterine body	History of postmenopausal bleeding
Carcinoma of breast	Examination
Carcinoma of prostate or rectum	Rectal examination
Visual defect	Test vision (near and distant)
Glaucoma	Schiotz tonometry
Coronary artery disease	Exercise ECG (optional) fasting cholesterol and triglycerides
Anaemia	Complete blood examination
Rheumatism	ESR
Obstructive airways disease	Spirometry (optional)
Reduced physical activity	History and counselling
Occupational problems	History and counselling

Consider these specific conditions in older middle-age:

Conditions	Manoeuvre
Hypothyroidism	Clinical examination in postmenopausal women
Menopause	Prescribe exogenous local or oral oestrogens
Primary open-angle glaucoma	Fundoscopy, visual field testing and measurement of intraocular pressure

important to their good health. Older people should remain active socially, avoid isolation and maintain ties with family members and friends. Community health and social organizations can facilitate group activities for older people, when possible, in community centres.

Immunization

Every year many older adults die or are incapacitated unnecessarily due to influenza or pneumonia. Older people can consult their physicians about immunization against these diseases.

Home safety

Falls are the leading cause of accidental injury and death among older adults. People and agencies responsible for housing for the elderly can provide such home safety measures as ample lighting, sturdy railings and steps, non-slip floor surfaces, and fire protection and detection measures.

Services to maintain independence

For those whose activity is limited, often relatively minor services can help older people maintain their independence. People should encourage programmes and services for: safe and affordable housing; dietary assistance through group meals and home meals; communications and transportation services; recreation and education opportunities; in-house services such as homemaker, visiting nurse and home health aides care; reading aids; and access to advice and services from appropriate health professionals. Home visiting by the doctor is essential to provide security for the elderly.

Age group 60–69

The frequency of routine physical checks will depend on the health and expected longevity of the patient. In the absence of any disease process or significant symptoms two year intervals may be sanctioned.

Health goals

To prolong physical, mental and social activity. To minimize the handicapping effect of the onset of chronic disease. To prepare for retirement, and bereavement.

Counselling

Changing lifestyle, nutrition, absence of family, reduction of income, and decreased physical activity.

Consider these specific conditions in the elderly:

Condition	Manoeuvre
Retirement distress	Final counselling examination before retirement as part of a series of periodic health examinations throughout adulthood
Progressive incapacity with ageing	Enquiry by doctor into physical, psychologic and social competence, conducted in the home, with organ-system enquiry and further action if indicated

Professional services

1. Full standard examination.
2. As for previous age group, especially to detect early signs of neoplastic or other chronic conditions.
3. Annual basic screening, influenza immunization, dental and foot care.
4. Other tests if indicated.

Age group 70–90

Consider these general issues:
The majority of people will have some problem under surveillance at this age. For those who are still in perfect health, a check-up every year gives them welcome reassurance. In the back of their minds they know that illness and death have sooner or later to be faced, and they want to renew acquaintance with the family doctor who will be such a tower of strength when this time comes.

Falls become an important predisposing cause of death. The interval between routine check-ups will be arranged between doctor and patient, and will vary according to the anxieties of either or both parties.

The important thing is for the routine check-up to be a time for general assessment of lifestyle, and an opportunity to encourage and to foster responsibility for health, mutual understanding and trust through counselling.

Health goals

1. To detect and distinguish disease from normal ageing, and where appropriate, treat.
2. To prevent avoidable misadventures (such as hypothermia, side-effects of drug treatment).
3. To educate patients and relatives in the changing physiology and needs of the aged.

4.   To preserve dignity and self-sufficiency for the patient with a framework of outside help which permits independence of mind if not of physique.

Problems

1.   Prevention is cure. Growing old is not preventable, but some medical problems of old age can be forestalled
e.g. painful feet→housebound lonely man→suicide
or broken glasses→fall→fractured hip.
Multiple pathology in the elderly.
      The elderly are often reluctant to report disabilities as they want to see themselves as healthy and therefore independent. Often they leave problems, obvious to others, to deteriorate to a point where their health is permanently damaged, or where those surrounding them are angered or alienated by their apparent pig-headedness. This is worse in the poorer and less well-educated (e.g. higher incidence of social class iv and v in presentation with acute retention with prostatic hyperplasia).

2.   Drugs and surgery may need extra caution if they are not to have unacceptably high physical, mental, social or ethical side-effects. If things are going wrong, consider stopping a drug rather than starting another.

3.   Isolation may be physical, social or emotional. Families may have moved away. Inflexible housing may create difficulties for the poorly mobile, and you will never know until a crisis occurs such as:

4.   Bereavement.

5.   Suicide, most common in older men.

6.   Retirement will be a crisis for a man or single woman, and the abrubt transition may be like a minor death. 'I'm in the way', 'I'm on the scrap heap now'. The retired may have no activities, no role, no status, and worst of all no money. Many are fit to work still, and some find their way back to employment with satisfaction.

7.   Families may need support to cope with a difficult relative.

8.   Resources are limited, both of the elderly and for their care.

Consider these general strategies:

Exercise

Regular physical activity for older adults can provide physical and psychological benefits, as well as help maintain flexibility and balance important to preventing falls. Older adults should therefore engage in exercise, such as daily walks, regularly. Dr Russell Gibbs' book 'Exercise for the over 50's' is a useful guide (Gibbs, 1980).

Nutrition

Older people have certain special dietary needs. Regular nutritious meals are important and particular care should be taken to include vegetables, sources of iron, calcium, and fibre, and use more fish, poultry, and legumes than red meat as sources of protein in the diet.

Preventive services

Some problems associated with ageing can be detected and corrected at an early state. Older adults should have health check-ups at least every two years until age 75, and every year thereafter. The following should be performed each time; blood pressure check (with follow-up and treatment, if warranted), hearing and vision examination, breast examination for women, urinalysis, and haematocrit. At less frequent intervals women should have Pap smears, and all should have stools examined for blood. When possible, these and other preventive services such as foot care, dental care and dietary guidance should be provided at a single location. Annual influenza immunization. Maintain tetanus immunity.

Medication

Older people frequently receive too much medication. Often fewer kinds of medications and lower dosages will suffice. Patients should ask their physicians to review regularly the medications they are taking. They should also request that medication be prescribed by its generic name, whenever feasible.

Events

As well as age-related health surveillance, the general practitioner may be allterted to *event related* preventive care.

It is difficult to encourage adults to look seriously at their equipment for dealing with stressful events that they have not yet experienced. Personal crises are events that happen to the family down the street, or are read about in the newspapers, with relative detachment. And yet when they do happen, they threaten mental health. Can we really prepare ourselves for those crises which beset everyone at some time in their lives?

Holmes and Rahe (1967) in the USA found that the ten most stressful areas were:

1. Death of a spouse
2. Divorce
3. Marital separation
4. Imprisonment

   5. Death of a close family member
   6. Personal illness
   7. Injury
   8. Marriage
   9. Being dismissed from work
  10. Changes in health of a family member.

Of course the authors are looking at events, rather than continual or recurring stress due to lifestyle processes, when individuals may have time to look at new options for dealing with it. However, failure to deal adequately with one crisis will certainly leave the individual at risk, and indicates a need to examine his coping skills and emotional equipment.

Dealing effectively with crisis requires adequate emotional equipment, the ability to adapt, and hopefully, sufficient social support. This social support involves one or more persons who are empathic, have good listening skills, and who have the ability to allow the afflicted person sufficient time to 'work through' both the factual and emotional areas of his stress.

The general practitioner is frequently called upon to provide this counselling. The general practitioner who has an ongoing doctor–patient relationship has the opportunity to offer preventive counselling and to promote appropriate social support networks for people under stress.

HEALTH PROMOTION COUNSELLING IN GENERAL PRACTICE

To meet the needs and expectations of his patients, today's doctor must assume many roles – healer, comforter, counsellor and educator – all of which demand time, devotion and teaching skills. He needs to be knowledgeable on health as well as disease, and to be able to trace disease to its cause(s). The best way to prevent disease is to promote health and a healthy way of life. Unfortunately, our disease-oriented medical education has not prepared doctors adequately for this role.

What can the busy general practitioner do to remedy this situation?

   1. Familiarize himself with health in its broadest aspects. Many excellent books are now available on this subject.

   2. Liaise with other health professionals, including the local community nurse, social worker, psychologist, clergyman, dietitian, dentist, health educator and teachers. Work with and learn from the team.

   3. Become aware of important environmental factors affecting the health of the local community (e.g. air and water pollution, food in school tuckshops, use of tobacco, alcohol and drugs, unhygienic practices, radiation hazards, etc.) and be prepared to say something about them.

4. Encourage responsible group programmes in the community (e.g. 5-Day Plans, Alcoholics Anonymous, Weight Watchers, GROW, fitness centres, etc.), by referring patients (or, at least, by not discouraging them through professional jealousy), and by becoming involved where possible.

5. Employ simple and inexpensive motivational and screening procedures appropriate to the age, sex and occupation of the individual (The Framingham Life Tables are available for this purpose).

6. Use every opportunity to educate patients. For example, while examining the breasts, teach self-examination techniques. Emphasize the limitations of medicine, for example, the uselessness of antibiotics for colds and viral infections. Noted Canadian physician, Sir William Osler, said, in 1920, 'One of the first duties of the physician is to educate the masses NOT to take medicine'.

7. Counsel patients, especially in regard to lifestyle, both individually and in small groups – the latter often being more effective and time-saving. The doctor should not underestimate his influence on patients. In the UK, about half of the people giving up smoking for health reasons, do so on the doctor's advice.

What can I, as a general practitioner, do to encourage my patient to promote his/her own health? How can I be an effective health counsellor? (Piggott, 1979).

1. Know how to be healthy yourself

It is a familiar taunt that many doctors are more interested in disease than they are in health.

We know a lot about how to be healthy. There are simple principles of good health and simple practices which promote health, and it is important to be aware of them.

*Eat a balanced diet with three regular meals, avoiding snacks.
*Learn to cope with stress and tension.
*Stay in shape with a sensible quota of regular exercise.
*Avoid cigarettes and encourage others to stop smoking.
*Drink alcohol in moderation or not at all.
*Get adequate and natural sleep.
*Understand the value of a positive attitude towards yourself, your job and your life.
*Develop rewarding personal relationships where you can discuss those things that matter most to you.
*Ensure satisfying sexual relationships.

2. *Know how you behave: model the behaviours you want to teach*

Who you are and what you do yourself are the strongest messages that come over to others. The old remark 'I cannot hear what you say for the thunder of what you do' is quite valid.

Your perception of your patient's health and the advice you give him, are both influenced by your own level of health. You are less likely to judge people to be overweight, if they are less obese than you. You are likely to feel your patient's alcohol consumption is acceptable provided it is less than yours. One study found that a larger proportion of non-smoking than currently smoking doctors advised all smoking patients to quit.

3. *See youself as being in the business of promoting your patient's health*

Most doctors have been trained to deal with sickness, their responsibility ending when their patients recover. In these circumstances, a patient in whom no pathology can be found is likely to be thought of as wasting the doctor's time. Unless you see yourself as being in the business of teaching your patient how to be healthy, it is unlikely that you will spend your time in this way.

4. *Believe in and have enthusiasm for health promotion*

Enthusiasm is infectious. If you are enthusiastic about promoting health, your patients are more likely to be enthusiastic too.

But don't become a health bore.

Health is a happy thing. Be serious about it by all means, but not solemn. Humour, and the perspective it gives, go a long way in education.

5. *Take an interest in how people learn and how to teach*

Some general practitioners are excellent teachers, but many are not. Little attention is given to teaching about the educational process in undergraduate courses.

This usually means that the only educational models doctors possess have come from their experiences at school and during their training. These are likely to be inappropriate.

Educational process is an area about which much is now known. It is important for doctors to be aware of the basic principles of both individual and group learning, if they wish to involve themselves in health education.

6. *Listen actively to your patient*

This means listening with the intention of understanding not only his words, but also his feelings, and being prepared to check with the patient that you are understanding him accurately.

7. Try to understand your patient's world and how he experiences it

Any help you give your patient is of limited use unless you have listened to him well enough to understand something of how he experiences his own world. He might differ from you in many ways, such as in age, education, social class, values, needs, responsibilities and experience. Because of this, 'advice' is usually inappropriate unless given in a context of helping the patient clarify his own situation and generate his own options. This is easily and frustratingly demonstrated when there is a wide cultural gap. Although masked, it applies in all situations. Dr Noburu Iwamura (Iwamura, 1978) reported on 17 years as a missionary general practitioner 'My goal has been to improve the health of the Nepali village people, yet I failed. Why? I failed because I used sophisticated technology brought from outside of the local culture. Being reminded that our Saviour Jesus came to live amongst the people, we should instead use his method.

'Here is a good example. He sent a missionary dietitian to Nepal. She went to a village and lived among the people, learning the local traditions and culture. Subsequently, she started a small village-level nutritional programme which was very successful. Why? Because she used the method of our living Saviour Jesus, allowing Him to work through her.

'The missionary dietitian built a simple grass hut where mothers from the village could bring their malnourished babies and learn how to make nutritious foods under the dietitian's guidance. This grass hut became very popular because it was fashioned after the cooking areas of the local village homes. Consequently, the mothers realized: "Yes, we can make such nutritious food in our own kitchens".

In addition, the missionary dietitian used (in instructing the women) only the traditional way of preparation, as well as locally available food. Each of the local kitchens was equipped with a stone mortar upon which the village women made their traditional wheat and corn flour. To this diet, the missionary simply added soy beans and demonstrated that a flour could also be made from the beans using the same mortar; a flour that was more nutritionally complete.

'Frequently, I saw a malnourished baby crying on the knee of a mother who was disappointed because she had failed to provide for her child. But once she was taught how to make nutritious food by her own hand with familiar tools and local resources, she was encouraged as she saw her child thriving with the supplemented diet. After three weeks of adequate nutrition, the child's improvement was remarkable.

'These successful mothers subsequently became the best health promoters in their communities. Having gained confidence in providing for their children and motivated by the Holy Spirit, they worked towards providing their neighbours with the same new-found skills and knowledge.

'The role of missionary medical workers is to learn an area's culture from the local people and then to clarify which aspects are harmful superstition and which are useful wisdom. They should then encourage the people to improve their lives using this traditional wisdom and available resources.

'When Jesus saw 5000 hungry people, he raised bread and fish from among the people in order to feed them. This is His method – for He uses resources from within a community to make a people self-reliant. To make people healthy, He uses us as His tools to motivate the proper use of local resources. The leader has been a great leader if, after the work is accomplished, the people say "we have done it ourselves".'

8.   Try to understand the meaning of your patient's behaviour within his culture and subculture

Also understand the meaning and acceptability of any behaviour he is expected to adopt.

9.   Take advantage of the opportunity offered by illness. Encourage your patient to ask himself: 'What is this illness saying about the way I'm living?'

An illness is a crisis for your patient. He can be especially ready at this time to review his behaviour and his values, and to decide to act in the future in a way more consistent with what is really important to him.

Doctors can learn the skills for helping their patients to think about these issues, grasping the 'teachable moment' when the patient is not sick, as in pregnancy:

'We are now more favourably placed to do effective preventive care in antenatal patient contacts than at any other time in recent history, and also at any time in the patient's life.

'Antenatal visits are the only long-established and well-understood preventive attendances by an otherwise well patient. Initially established on negative principles, that is, to detect complications, these visits also can be used for positive contributions to health education.

'Patients are eager to learn when pregnant. If personal and social circumstances are favourable, their motivation is at its peak for learning positive health and lifestyles which will provide optimum conditions in the new baby's home' (Fredman, 1979).

10.   Treat your patient's underlying needs with respect

Don't expect him to give up a behaviour unless he has some way of meeting the needs that prompt that behaviour.

Your patient's current behaviour can be seen as part of his present way of dealing with the demands of his daily life.

To attempt to change a behaviour without understanding its role in your patient's life makes little sense and is not likely to achieve much.

The important task is to help your patient find better ways of handling things than that of adopting health damaging practices.

*11. The general practitioner has a key role to play in health promotion by being available **and offering continuing support**.*

Let me quote from Zifferblatt and Wilbur (Zifferblatt and Wilbur, 1977):

'The major obstacle today in reducing cardiovascular morbidity and mortality is not the physician's ability to get initial changes in patient behaviour, but that of obtaining long-lasting change . . .

'Evidence from several long-term clinical trials strongly suggests that a patient's ability to establish long-lasting behaviour changes depends more on the sensitive, empathic and continuous manner in which any reasonable treatment is employed, rather than on any unique aspect of the treatment itself . . .

'To maintain a new change, a person must continually confront and resolve the problems caused by personal and environmental factors, such as work schedules, social situations, and family conflicts. Such changes, tantamount to lifestyle changes, may require time and the aid of a supportive and consistent clinic environment. Unfortunately, most attempts to change health behaviour are limited to short time periods. Short-term training influences are usually no match for the multitude of factors that affect the person's behaviour in the weeks, months, and years to come.'

Prepare to provide continual support for the patient over time. Unlike counselling sessions, problems with health behaviour do not occur on a regular schedule. It may be impossible to schedule clinic visits more than once or twice per month, but it is very important to have more frequent contact by telephone or mail, especially during the early stages of a programme.

It is important to tackle problems soon after they occur, rather than letting the patient report a long period of failure and frustration at the next counselling session. Moreover, a patient's initial enthusiasm for change often drops very rapidly, and, to help maintain commitment, the patient needs support and encouragement.

If the clinician or members of his or her staff can frequently demonstrate an interest in a patient's problems and progress, this will provide an invaluable contribution to a successful programme.

The doctor should seek the active participation of a patient's family in all aspects of a health change programme. The support and encouragement of family and friends is necessary for lasting change, and, clearly, a successful health maintenance programme involving diet requires the full cooperation of the family member(s) who purchase and prepare household foods.

To support already functioning local groups, or to develop self-help groups in your practice, focusing on weight control, relaxation and stress management, smoking cessation, parenting skills and so on, can be a direct extension of the doctor's health promotion role.

12.   Transfer the skills, knowledge and attitudes your patient will need to promote his own health

*General concepts that are important in understanding how the body works and how to be healthy.
*Infectious diseases, resistance and immunization.
*Healthy eating and drinking.
*Healthy activity.
*How to handle stress and how to relax.
*Getting to know yourself better (becoming clearer about your interests, strengths, values, goals).
*Making friends and having good relationships with other people.
*Making it more fun to live in your family.
*Alcohol.
*Smoking.
*Health and your workplace.
*Preventing accidents.
*Being out of work: retirement from 17 to 70.
*How to have a say in matters that affect your environment and your health.
*How you have come to fall ill.
*Mutually satisfying sexual activity.

The task is to teach the most important things about each topic in the simplest and clearest way, with the emphasis on things that your patient can actually do to promote his own health (Allen, 1977).

In working out how to do this, it is useful to ask about each topic: 'If my patient is to be able to promote his own health,

What skills are involved?
What knowledge is necessary?
What attitudes are desirable?'

Some are not difficult to transfer. However, in order to be successful in teaching many of them, the doctor will be at a considerable disadvantage unless he has come to understand something of how people learn and how to teach.

A good way for him to learn these things is to experience personally effective teaching of these skills, knowledge and attitudes, with himself as the 'learner' in specially devised workshops.

13.   Keep informed on a wide range of resources which could be useful to your patients

In order to give your patient access to a wide range of options, you must first be aware yourself of what these options are.

The range of people, organizations and opportunities that could be helpful to your patient has very much expanded in recent years. Keeping up with them requires a deliberate effort.

14.   The general practitioner has a role to play outside the consulting room, by **influencing the environment**

Ask: What messages does my practice give about how to be healthy? i.e. What is my clinic's 'hidden curriculum'?

Is the place cheerful? Are patients expected to sit in rooms in which others smoke? Is literature on how to be healthy provided for people while they are waiting? Are there educational posters, thoughtfully placed? What are the furnishings saying about our attitude toward patients?

The staff – are they overweight? Do they smoke? Are they chronically tired? How are their relationships with each other? Do they seem interested in health and being healthy?

What about the food served to patients and sold in the hospital canteen? Are we proud of the model it offers for healthy nutrition?

Have patients the opportunity of drinking cool water or fresh fruit juices, or are there only heavily-sweetened fruit juices or sugar-laden cordials, with soft drink machines and cigarette and confectionary dispensers out there in the lobby for visitors?

Will hospital patients go home with an idea of what really healthy food looks and tastes like as a result of their stay?

How much concern is shown about how patients came to be ill, and how they can promote their own health in the future?

15.   Be concerned about the effect of your patient's work on his health

In an impressive fifteen year study of ageing, the strongest predictor of longevity was 'work satisfaction'. The second best predictor was overall self-rated 'happiness'. These two sociopsychological factors predicted longevity better than a rating by an examining doctor of physical functioning, or a measure of the use of tobacco, or genetic inheritance. Controlling these other variables statistically did not alter the dominant role of work satisfaction (Palmore, 1969). The ill-health implications of long-term unemployment have been found to be considerable.

Try to understand what your patient's job involves and what it must be like to do his work every day.

'I work in a chocolate factory' might sound like the fulfilment of a childhood dream. But it could hide a picture of repetitious work with an unpleasant foreman under noisy and physically stressful conditions.

If there are major industries in your area, make the time to visit them. If you see a patient made sick by his working environment, help him to think through the steps he can take to do something about it. If the situation warrants it, be prepared to do something yourself. You could talk to the occupational health nurse or directly to the management about what you have noticed. You could discuss it with the division of occupational health and radiation control, or let the environmental section of your health authority know about it.

16.   Exert your personal influence for health promotion through local councils, schools, letters to the editor and so on

Threats to health are often slow to be recognized, and the community depends on those with special expertise to bring them to attention.

Speak out. If you won't raise questions publicly about matters that affect health, who will?

17.   The ballot box: ask your local candidates to explain their positions on health issues

Politicians respond to public concern and pressure. If voters are not concerned about health issues, why shoud politicians be losing sleep about them?

You are in a better position than most to ask the relevant questions, to judge the adequacy of replies that are given, and to draw public attention to the health implications of the policies that are being pursued.

Beyond the health-related aspects of the face-to-face relationships at work and play, stand the *structural, social* and *economic* factors which promote ill-health.

The epidemics of road deaths and serious injuries, of the many stress-related diseases, including the cigarette and alcohol diseases, of obesity, of dental caries and so on, are increasingly being recognized as the unwelcome but inevitable by-products of the indiscriminate and frenzied pursuit of economic growth. Instead of producing the goods we really need – and the goods that will last – we make more inessential goods, and we actually plan their rapid obsolescence. Similarly, in producing and transporting inessential goods we generate accidents and create more health hazards from industrial pollutants. We go on producing damaging products like cigarettes, and over-refined foods like fibre-deficient white flour, and entice people to consume the alcoholic drinks which promote physical and interpersonal distress (Draper *et al.*, 1976).

Prevention has to be directed at the underlying causes, rather than focusing mistakenly on symptoms, and expressing useless exhortations. For example, essentially moralistic and puritanical appeals to individuals to 'pull your socks up', to modify their personal life and so on, achieve little, and distract attention from the policies and practices which generate the stresses and risks. Attention has to be directed to remove or reduce the conditions which pressure people to lead unhealthy lives.

Let us stop pretending there is any cure in high moral precepts. Good advice has been preached too long to men and women who have to survive in the best manner they can. Preaching merely increases the strain which they have not been able to bear, it increases the self-criticism of the conscientious, and disheartens and provokes rejection from the majority of people because it widens the gap between their ideals and their reality, without giving them the power to approach 'living wisely'.

What can be done? One approach, once the present conflict between the pursuit of indiscriminate economic growth and public health is widely recognized, is to develop economic, social and health policies in an integrated way, rather than putting profits first and thus creating health and social problems. The solution to these problems lies in the creation of appropriately human technology rather than the expensive and complex technology which often squanders energy, creates unemployment, and thereby leads to anxiety states, depression, alcoholism and the like.

The integrated approach is summarized well in a study document by the Christian Medical Commission (Kingma, 1976) Kingma, S.J.: 'Seeds of Health', a Study Guide. Christian Medical Commission, World Council of Churches, Geneva, 1976.

A COMMUNITY APPROACH

'More and more health workers around the world are learning that health care in the form of curative services and institutions is very inadequate. Its impact on the health and well-being of the communities served is measured only in terms of restoring those who fall ill. This is true even if hospital services are coupled with a 'rural outreach' programme or include family planning services and the care of chronic diseases such as tuberculosis. The fact is that each patient represents a failure of society to prevent that episode of sickness. The problems are especially severe among the poor and rural people of developing countries where most sickness and death results from nutritional and communicable diseases – preventable problems. This is a total community problem. To come to grips with it means taking a completely new look at the whole community. To make a substantial impact on health, efforts in the medical and health sector must be viewed as just one part of total community development, human development. They must involve the people themselves in the development process and in learning to care for themselves.

'The International Development Research Centre of Ottawa, Canada, has released a film entitled *Rural Health Workers*. This 25 minute colour film (16 mm) examines six health programmes in different parts of the world where attempts are made to bridge the gap between sophisticated city hospitals and the small rural communities where health services are often non-existent. In examining these six examples, the film demonstrates that there is no one way to meet the health needs of rural peoples living in different situations. It further demonstrates the imagination and involvement of the rural people themselves in countries as diverse as Panama, Thailand, Canada, Bangladesh, Iran and Venezuela. The film is available with English or French soundtrack.

'The Chimaltenango Development Project is one example of an effective approach to health care and total development, the type of care which is an example of primary preventive health care now being encouraged by the World Council of Churches/Christian Medical Commission and the World Health Organization. It is only one answer to the problem, a method which seems to be appropriate in the highlands of Guatemala. Two thirds of the population of this country consists of Indians – most of them living in poverty. Over 80% of the arable land is owned by 2% of the population as well as by large foreign-based corporations. Nearly 50% of the Indian children born alive die before reaching the age of five. Malnutrition is a major problem because those Indians who do own land are often not able to grow enough to feed their families from one harvest to the next. The struggle for health is thus a lifelong struggle for food and water!

'When Dr Carrol Berhorst first came to Guatemala, he came to set up a mission hospital. It quickly became obvious to him that a curative institution could do very little about the root causes of disease and misery. So he made a major effort to get to know the people and to find out what they thought they needed. This was their priority list of problems to be solved: social injustice, abuse of land tenure, population problems, poor agricultural marketing and production, widespread malnutrition, inadequate health training, and lack of curative services related to their needs. In order to have the greatest impact on the health problems of this area, it was necessary to develop a programme which had several related aspects, each focusing on a different type of activity.

'The first initiative was the training of health promoters. These were members of the Indian community who were trained in a simple fashion to treat certain symptoms of disease with a relatively small and basic supply of drugs. They were elected by a local health committee from each village. While their activities were initially oriented to curative practice, they also promoted community self-confidence and encouraged the Indians to assume even greater control of their own lives. They were able to stimulate community thinking about common problems and to assist in the discovery of ways for improving their situation.

'A training programme was then initiated to prepare a group of workers whose task would be in the area of agricultural and community work. In teaching hygiene, nutrition and modern agricultural methods, these workers were able to complement the health promoter's work. They encouraged the cooperative efforts of groups of farmers. A revolving loan fund was set up for cooperating groups of farmers to assist them in securing improved seeds, fertilizer and other items.

'Another activity was the Simajuleu water project. By cooperative efforts the Indians tapped into a spring and transferred the water by means of a pipeline to the village several kilometers away. The benefits of safe drinking water have been quickly realized.

'Since land ownership is a crucial factor in causing hunger, a land foundation was formed. It has been able to negotiate with certain land owners for the purchase of land which is then distributed as plots among the farmers of a given district. This purchase is repaid by the farmers themselves out of the yield from their harvest.

'Improved agricultural techniques have increased yields, making the repayment of the loan relatively easy.

'The original clinic has grown into a small hospital. It serves as a referral centre for the health promoters when they identify illnesses which are beyond their capacity. It is also the centre for the ongoing training of health promoters and agricultural extensionists. In addition, this hospital is unusual in its approach to patient care. The staff believes that the patients themselves should establish the terms on which they will be treated. One of these terms is that hospitalization shall not isolate the patient from his or her family and community. The patient's family cooks and cares for him and thus the hospital atmosphere reflects the local living style. Feeling more at home, the patient is much more capable of waging his own mental fight against disease.

'This project has demonstrated the capacity to promote self-reliance and to assist the Cakchiquee Indians in improving the dignity of their lives!'

A film of this project has been produced by the World Council of Churches and Teldok Films, and is available in English, Spanish, French and German. For further information contact – Christian Medical Commission, World Council of Churches, 150 Route de Ferney, 1211 Geneva 20, Switzerland.

BASIC ISSUES IN HEALTH AND DISEASE

This project is illustrative of one style of primary health care in the context of community development. Its importance, however, goes beyond that. It has been able to highlight some of the most fundamental issues in the health and well-being of a rural community. What are some of these basic determinants of health (and disease), and how can they be viewed in the wider context of other less developed countries' needs for promoting health?

1. Water, food and sanitation: At one level, these are major factors in the degree of health experienced by a community. Their importance cannot be overemphasized. Adequate provision of safe drinking water and the effective use of simple sanitation will do more for a reduction in morbidity and mortality than many other types of effort – certainly more than a purely curative medical programme by itself. The same can be said for nutrition. The role of undernutrition and protein wasting in eroding communal and individual health is extensive, affecting the success of breast feeding, childhood growth and development, adult productivity, and many other aspects.

Often, measures in support of adequate food, water and sanitation are postponed while a medical service is established to meet the 'obvious needs'. Besides, health workers find the food and water shortage a difficult one and outside their capacity. The classic responses of teaching the universal boiling of water and importing quantities of protein-rich food have inherent limitations with shortages of fuel and money, and cannot be long-term solutions. What then are the answers? To begin with, total community development needs to take its rightful place as a primary effort in health promotion. An appropriate style of technology, and an infra-structure in the area of agriculture and community organization is essential.

However, it must be understood that this kind of exercise to assist people in need only begins to touch the basic issues. The impact on health will still be limited unless two further dimensions of the problem are con-sidered.

2.   *Social justice:* Any effort to address the poverty and food problem at the most basic level will quickly encounter the questions of maldistribution of community services, employment opportunities, land tenure and social injustice. These inevitably are political problems. It must be frankly said that poverty and lack of food and the inaccessibility of health services are generally NOT problems of scarcity, but of distribution, control and power (Sider, 1977). The precise profile of the root causes will differ from country to country, of course. But, where health is concerned, the basic issues are to be found at this level, in industrial and less developed countries alike. Planning that makes a real difference to the health of the community must analyse cause and effect until the essential causes at the level of money and power are identified. This is as true for smaller scale efforts of voluntary agencies as it is for governments. The honesty and courage exhibited by the people of Chimaltenango have shown that change can take place.

3.   *Health planning as if people mattered:* All of the best expertise and planning for health development that regards the 'target population' as 'recipients' of a 'delivery system' will simply perpetuate an injustice of another kind. It will ignore the right of people to participate with dignity in their lives. Participation of people in the identification of needs, in the setting of priorities, in planning, in implementation and in control of their own health care is emerging in many places as a dynamic factor of great importance. The patterns of isolation, resignation and dependence are so well established, that a motivational process will be required in many communities and societies. The fact is however, that *people* are the greatest existing resource for health (not the burgeoning medical technology which is primarily restorative), and their potential is maximized when the health care system 'belongs' to them. This thrust is seen in some of the emerging terminology in health planning: 'the demystification of health technology', 'the democratization of health', 'be your own MD', 'self-reliance in health', and the like. It is also reflected in the entire concept of primary preventive health care as articulated by the World Health Organization. The necessity for this approach is clear. People can no longer be excluded from health planning (Kingma, 1976).

People participating in health planning

How can we involve people in the health planning process to secure the expression by the entire community of its needs, and the priorities to be set within those needs? What steps are necessary to mobilize the community for its maximum involvement in all stages of the programme? This is the focus of this final section which outlines resources for learning further about strategies for the planning dialogue in the community.

Much has been written over the past few years about the necessary components of primary health care, or community health care. Among these, the participation of people in the planning process in identifying needs, setting priorities, and carrying out the programme, has long been recognized by health planners and development planners to be perhaps the most essential. The questions remain: 'How does one secure the expression of the entire community of its needs, and the priorities to be set within those needs?'

A very practical outline of the steps necessary to develop a community health programme has been written by Mary Johnston, based on more than ten years' experience in the Dana Sehat programme in Central Java, Indonesia. This considerable experience is apparent in the careful working out of the approach she has presented. The Dana Sehat programme is based on the concept of a community development programme, built upon a health insurance scheme. 'Dana Sehat', literally translated, means 'health funds'.

Beginning around the city of Solo, the programme has been expanded to include many communities and small hamlets in Indonesia, and incorporates a wide variety of development activities including cooperatives, credit unions and sanitary measures. Further details on the Dana Sehat programme can be found in the article by Dr. Gunawan Nugroho in the WHO book, *Health by the People*, 1975, as well as Mary Johnston's article from *Contact, Issue 43*, the summary from which is quoted here.

'Summary:

Major steps in developing a community health programme:

1. Promotion with the government.
2. Consolidation of the health staff.
3. Approach to the community.
4. Social preparation of the community.
5. Field preparation.
   5.1. Selection of initial project area.
   5.2. Collection of data about the community.
   5.3. Determination of problems to be tackled and setting priorities.
   5.4. Planning programme implementation.
6. Implementation of the programme.
7. Monitoring.
8. Assessment.

9.   Revision.
10.   Expansion of the established programme.
11.   Extension of the programme to other communities.
12.   Promotion and training in new areas, and repeat of the whole
      process in a new community.'

One lesson emerging from this experience was presented in a recently
published report on the programme, summarized as follows: 'Success
depended on such factors as correct timing in the presentation of ideas and
adequate social preparation. Social preparation involved not only the
dissemination of information and explanations about the purpose and
aims of the scheme but, of even greater importance, the encouragement of
the people themselves to participate actively and assume responsibility for
the scheme. Cooperation with government services is essential for healthy
growth of a community programme. This cooperation is with village
leaders and with appropriate government services at the district level . . .
or possibly even higher.'

Readers who wish to explore the practice management implications of
participatory community health programmes are referred to *Contact, Issue
43*, February 1978, published by the Christian Medical Commission,
World Council of Churches, 150 Route de Ferney, 1211 Geneva 20,
Switzerland.

Among the concerns that are often voiced by those involved in health
care planning is one which can be summed up in the phrase: 'Let's make
the most of the lessons we have already learned. The wheel may not yet be
perfect, but it has been invented.' Dr. Rufino L. Macagba, Jr. of the
Health Care Systems of World Vision International believes that the last
two decades have not only provided many rational guidelines which can
now be applied to the health planning process, but also that there are time-
proven principles of management that can be brought to bear on the
administration of health programmes. His book *Health Care Guidelines*, for
use in developing countries, seeks to present a simplified course in
management for key people leading health projects or community health
teams. It encompasses many of the same concerns as Mary Johnston
presents in *Contact, Issue 43*, with a good deal more stress on the organizational and management aspects, in the effort to promote wider application
of care with existing resources. This paperback book has 111 pages and is
priced at US$ 4.00 plus postage and 10% handling charges. *Health Care
Guidelines* can be otained from: Evangelical Missionary Alliance, 19
Draycott Place, London SW3 2SJ, England; or MARC, 919 West Hun-
tington Drive, Monrovia, California 91016, USA.

Finally, in considering practice management for health promotion,
doctors need to consider whether community development efforts will be
enough. In some circumstances, radical political change, including land
reforms and redistribution of control of the means of production will be
necessary to provide minimal nutritional and health needs for all the

people (Fanon, 1961). Sometimes it may be necessary to follow the example of Dr Che Guevara, who left his practice, and joined in the struggle for social and political justice as a precondition for health for the majority of people in his country.

At an international level, the threat of war, especially nuclear war, confronts doctors with perhaps the greatest threat to the health of the people. The whole fragile earth is threatened by this rush toward nuclear suicide. Nuclear disarmament is a global concern for which we doctors must play our part.

References

1. McCamy, J.C. and Presley, J. (1975). *Human Life Styling* Harper and Row Publishers, New York, Hagerstown, San Francisco, London. Wright H.B. (ed.) (1976). *A Longer Life*. Blackie & Son (Glasgow: Blackie) Vol. 1. 'Basic Health Maintenance'; Vol. 2. 'Heart Disease'; Vol. 3. 'Fitness Without Fantasies'; Vol. 4. 'A Woman's Life'
2. Piggott, R. (1979). *Personal Communication*. In writing this chapter I have drawn on roneod papers 'Health Professionals as Health Promoters: Ideas/Opportunies/Options' and 'Education for Self Responsibility: A Coordinating Concept for Health Education' by Robert Piggott, Health Commission of New South Wales, Australia, and quoted a number of passages from these with permission
3. American Heart Association (1973). *Coronary Risk Handbook: estimating risk of coronary heart disease in daily practice.* (New York: American Heart Association)
4. Robbins, L.C. and Hall, J.H. (1970). *How to Practice Prospective Medicine.* Methodist Hospital of Indiania, Indianopolis. Also Beeson, L. and Phillips, R. (1977) *Procedure Manual for Health Age Appraisal.* (Loma Linda, California: School of Health)
5. LaDou, J., Sherwood, J.N. and Hughes, L. (1975). Health hazard appraisal in patient counseling. *West. J. Med.,* **122** 177–80.
6. Belloc, N.B. and Breslow, L. (1972). Relationships of physical health status and health practices. *Preventive Med.,* **1**, 409–21.
7. Table reprinted with permission from Allen, D.W. (1979). Preventive care in general practice. *Austr. Family Phys.,* **8**, 1124
8. Marx, M.B., Barnes, G., Somers, G.W. and Garrity, T.F. (1978). The health script: its relationship to illness in a college population. *Transact. Anal. J.,***8**, 339
9. Further details are available in the whole prevention issue of *Austr. Family Phys.,* **8**, 219–323. Doctors will be well rewarded for detailed study of Spitzer, W.O. *et al.*, The Periodic Health Examination. *Can. Med. Assoc.,* **121**, 1193–1254. Copies of this report and the monograph may be obtained from Health Services Directorate, Tunney's Pasture, Ottawa, Ontario KIA 1BA, Canada.
10. Cormack, J., Marinker, M. and Morrell, D. (eds.) (1976). *Practice: A Handbook of Primary Medical Care.* (London: Kluwer–Harrap Handbooks)
11. Royal Australian College of General Practitioners (1977). *RACGP Health Record System*, RACGP, Melbourne.

12. Carson, S. (1979). *A Manual for General Practice*. Australian Edition, Beecham Research Laboratories, Melbourne. U.K. Edition, Beecham Research Laboratories, Brentford.
13. Cullen, K. (1975). *Prevention of Emotional Disorders in Pre-school Children*. Family Medicine Programme, RACGP, Melbourne.
14. Gibbs, R. (1980). *Exercise for the Over 50's* (Sunbooks)
15. Iwamura, N. (1978). Personal Communication included in the *Proceedings of the Sixth International Congress of Christian Medical Students, Davos*.
16. Fredman, R.M. (1979). Antenatal preventive care. *Austr. Family Phys.*, **8**, 227
17. Zifferblatt, S. and Curtis, W. (1977). Maintaining a healthy heart: guidelines for a feasible goal. *Prevent. Med.* **6**, 514
18. Allen, D.W. (1977). *Total Health Syllabus*. 2nd edition, First Australian Institute of Total Health.
19. Palmore, E. (1969). Predicting longevity: a follow-up controlling for age. *Gerontologist*, **9**, 247
20. Draper, P., Best, G. and Dennis, J. (1976). *Health, Money and the National Health Service*. Unit for the Study of Health Policy, Guy's Hospital Medical School, London
21. For further study of this subject, see Sider, R. (1977). *Rich Christians in an Age of Hunger*. Paulist Press, New Jersey
22. Kingma, S.J., *Seeds of Health, a Study Guide*. Christian Medical Commission, World Council of Churches, Geneva, 1976, quoted with permission.
22. Fanon, F. (1961). *The Wretched of the Earth*. (New York: Grove Press)

For further study of the community health dimension, readers are referred to the World Health Organization series 'Health for All'.

No. 1 –Alma-Ata 1978: Primary Health Care (1978).

No. 2 –Formulating Strategies for Health for All by the Year 2000 (1979).

No. 3 –Global Strategy for Health for All by the Year 2000 (1981).

No. 4 –Development of Indicators for Monitoring Progress Towards Health for All by the Year 2000 (1981).

No. 5 –Managerial Process for National Health Development: Guiding Principles (1981).

No. 6 –Health Programme Evaluation: Guiding Principles (1981).

No. 7 –Plan of Action for Implementing the Global Strategy for Health for All and Index to the 'Health for All' Series, No. 1–7 (1982).

6

Principles of Management in Patient Care

SELWYN CARSON (NEW ZEALAND)

In the community, there is a need for good sensible doctoring, good general practice. The problem is to look after people in the traditional manner yet, at the same time, deliver the developing medical technology. A simple, problem orientated system of practice records plus guidelines for technical care, make a simple technical pattern for practice, leaving the doctor to get on with his real job: caring, listening and being available. It is possible for the solo GP to do this as well as the doctor in a group practice.

Primary health care services should be patient-orientated, flexible, and suited to each local community, for the needs of each local community are different. Decentralization and autonomy of local services is desirable, but is more difficult to achieve in urban areas overshadowed by base hospitals, which are attuned to academic and professional needs rather than patient needs, than it is in small towns where the local hospital is staffed by GPs and is close to the people.

Part of the GP's expertise is to know the range of services that can be of use to his patients and to see that they are accessible when they are needed. The GP, himself, should be accessible and available when **he** is needed. A doctor who offers a fine preventive health service, but who is not available should a child have a middle ear infection or a patient be in pain, is not much use to the patient. It follows that the practice should not be bigger than one can cope with, and there should be good communication between the patient and the doctor. On the other hand, preventive health care is also just as much the role of the general practitioner as is emergency care. The practice nurse can be of great help both in emergencies and first aid and also in routine tasks such as the surveillance of children, preventive health care in all age groups, and preventive maintenance care in high-incidence chronic illness. There is always so much more that the GP can do. The intelligent use of other health professionals can increase his effectiveness.

It is of use to have protocols, where possible, for both emergency and preventive care, and a start has been made to set these down (Carson, 1975). It is emphasized that any protocols should be mere guidelines and flexible for use in different situations. The actual services will be dictated by the patient needs as the doctor and patient see them.

OBSTETRICS

Routine antenatal care is usually performed best by GPs and the technical, physical care is usually good in developed countries. Adequate nutrition, the correction of defects where possible, the prevention of toxaemia, the management of blood incompatibility, and the anticipation of fetal abnormalities and difficulties in delivery are all part of the routine technology; and practice nurses, with a midwifery background, can be of great use to the patient and the doctor. Now, attention is being paid not only to education in the anatomy and physiology of pregnancy, but also to the personal quality of the antenatal and birth experience for the patient and the family. These aspects are not as well defined as the physical ones, but it seems possible to overcome ignorance and the fear of childbirth, to aid the emotional health of the mother and family, and to foster early bonding between the mother and the child (Cullen, 1976). There is no doubt that breast feeding is best and the involvement of the husband or partner is desirable in antenatal preparation.

Postnatal care includes family planning and contraception, a simple, technical subject, rich in family dynamics, that should be included in the shared expertise of the health team. Not the least of the knowledge available and able to be set down is that of the iatrogenic illnesses caused by unwise medication.

Protocols will vary in different countries. Examples of those used for routine obstetric care in New Zealand at present are to be found on pp. 93–7.

Routine obstetric care (see Figures 1–8)

NEONATAL CARE

If there is an enthusiastic practice nurse with midwifery training, and she can visit the patient at home after discharge from hospital, then so much the better. The most helpful situation occurs when the same professionals are concerned in antenatal care, the delivery and home visiting after the birth.

Examples of useful guidelines, for routine neonatal care, again designed for New Zealand are to be found on pp. 99–103.

INFANT CARE

The service our infant patients get is usually fragmented, overlapping and uncoordinated. This has increased with the need to deliver more techno-

Routine Obstetric Care

Consultation Plan

DATE	DOCTOR	PRACTICE STAFF
Initial. About 8 weeks pregnant	X	X
12 weeks pregnant	X	X
16 weeks pregnant	X	X
20 weeks pregnant	X	X
24 weeks pregnant	X	X
28 weeks pregnant	X	X
32 weeks pregnant	X	X
34 weeks pregnant	X	X
36 weeks pregnant	X	X
37 weeks pregnant	X	X
38 weeks pregnant	X	X
39 weeks pregnant	X	X
Birth	X	
6 weeks Post-Natal	X	X

A1

Figure 1   Consultation plan

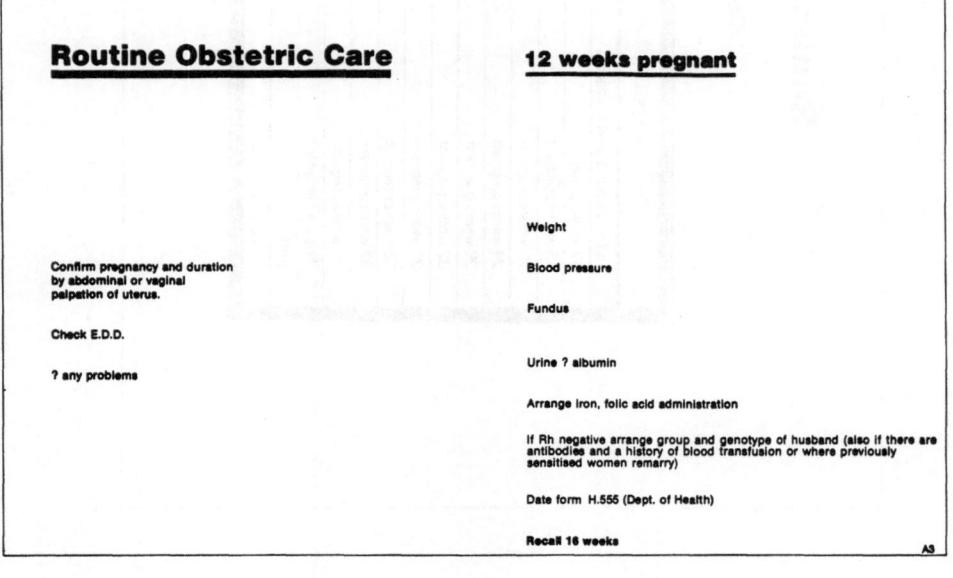

Routine Obstetric Care

Initial (about 8 weeks pregnant)

Well woman examination (see page C2) with special attention to pelvis and breasts

Estimate E.D.D.

Decide most suitable hospital

? any problems

High Risk Patients May Include:
Elderly primigravida
Grand multipara
Those with a bad obstetric history
Where there is a previous history of LSCS
Hypertension
Short stature
Diabetes
Obesity
Other diseases e.g. tuberculosis, cardiac problems
Social problems e.g. solo parent, ethnic cultures.

Well woman questionnaire with special attention to obstetric history (see page C1)

Arrange also: Antenatal blood screen (including full antibody screen Groups I and II)

On mass X-Ray form note patient is pregnant

Arrange hospital booking

Prepare form H.555 (Dept. of Health) and attach to patient's records

Recall 12 weeks

A2

Figure 2   The initial consultation (about 8 weeks pregnant)

Routine Obstetric Care

12 weeks pregnant

Confirm pregnancy and duration by abdominal or vaginal palpation of uterus.

Check E.D.D.

? any problems

Weight

Blood pressure

Fundus

Urine ? albumin

Arrange iron, folic acid administration

If Rh negative arrange group and genotype of husband (also if there are antibodies and a history of blood transfusion or where previously sensitised women remarry)

Date form H.555 (Dept. of Health)

Recall 16 weeks

A3

Figure 3   12 weeks pregnant

Routine Obstetric Care   **32 weeks pregnant**

Weight

Blood pressure

Fundus. Record girth measurement.

Foetal position, foetal heart

Confirm foetal position and
foetal heart   Urine ? albumin

Check E.D.D.   Encourage iron, folic acid, fluoride administration

Where there is a bad history arrange
base-line oestriol and ? weekly oestriols.   Encourage care of breasts

Confirm physiotherapy

? any problems

Rh negative woman, Rh positive husband,
administer 1 ml anti-D globulin, intramuscular

Date form H.555 (Dept. of Health)

Recall 34 weeks   A8

Figure 4   32 weeks pregnant

Routine Obstetric Care   **6 weeks post-natal**

	Mother	**Baby**
Examine breasts and pelvis	Weight	Routine examination infant age 6 weeks (See page B4)
Cervical smear	Blood pressure	
? contraception	Temperature	**Recall age 3 months**
? any problems	Encourage breast feeding, iron, fluoride administration	
? follow up e.g. bacteriuria ? I.V.P. hypertension	Encourage exercises for abdominal and pelvic muscles.	
	Discuss adequate diet, rest and personal care	
	Date form H.555 (Dept. of Health) and patient signs	A15

Figure 5   6 weeks postnatal

Possible Adverse Effects in the Human Foetus and Neonate Attributed to Maternally Administered Drugs

Drug class	Agent	Possible foetal or neonatal effect	Drug class	Agent	Possible foetal or neonatal effect
Drugs acting on CNS	Strong analgesics (narcotics)	Neonatal depression "Withdrawal symptoms"	Antimicrobial agents	Anticoagulants	? Foetal and neonatal haemorrhage
	Mild analgesics (salicylates)	Transient coagulation defects		Aminoglycosides (streptomycin); kanamycin; gentamicin	Ototoxicity
	Barbiturates	Neonatal depression Increased rate of neonatal drug metabolism Foetal asphyxia (if maternal hypotension induced by barbiturate)		Tetracyclines	Abnormal dentition Maternal hepatotoxicity Renal toxicity
	Local anaesthetics	Foetal bradycardia Neonatal depression Maternal hypotension (spinal anaesthesia) Methaemoglobinaemia (prilocaine)		Chloramphenicol	Cardiovascular collapse, 'gray syndrome'
				Sulphonamides	Neonatal kernicterus Haemolytic anaemia in those with G6PD deficiencies (rare)
	Phenothiazines	Neonatal sedation ? Retinopathy (high doses) Extrapyramidal reactions		Trimethoprim	Anti-folate effects
				Nitrofurantoin	Haemolytic anaemia in those with G6PD deficiencies (rare)
Drugs acting on hormonally regulated processes	Anticonvulsants benzodiazepines phenytoin	Neonatal depression Congenital abnormalities	Drugs acting on cardiovascular system	Antimalarials quinine chloroquine	Thrombocytopenia Retinopathy Ototoxicity
	Antithyroid agents iodides (NB cough mixtures) radio-iodine propylthiouracil, carbimazole	Foetal euthyroid goitre Severe hypothyroidism in foetus Foetal goitre		β-Adrenergic receptor blockers	Neonatal depression
				Antihypertensives reserpine	Nasal stuffiness, lethargy
				magnesium sulphate	Neuromuscular weakness, lethargy
	Hypoglycaemic agents	? Prolonged hypoglycaemia	Antineoplastic agents	thiazides	? Thrombocytopenia
	Androgens and certain progestagens	Virilisation of female		Cytotoxic drugs	Congenital abnormalities
	Oestrogens	Feminisation of male Adenocarcinoma of cervix in children	Miscellaneous	Nicotine	Small for dates babies Increased perinatal mortality
	Corticosteroids	? Congenital abnormalities Increased risk of prematurity and/or intra-uterine growth retardation ? Adrenal crisis on withdrawal (theroretically possible)		Cannabis	
				LSD	Foetal malformations
				Water-soluble Vit K	Neonatal jaundice

From "Drug Effects on the Foetus" Singh & Minkin N.E. and M.P., November 1973.

Figure 6　Possible adverse effects in the human fetus and neonate attributed to maternally administered drugs

Breast Care during Pregnancy

1. Throughout the pregnancy a well fitting bra will help prevent loss of breast shape.

2. No breast care is necessary in the first 6 months of pregnancy.

3. In the last 3 months it is not necessary to use soap on the breasts. The skin secretes protectivie oil which will strengthen the nipples and make them supple. Pure lanoline is a good ointment.

4. To desensitise the nipples can be rubbed gently daily with a towel or the nipples can be pulled out gently several times a day.

5. If the nipples are flat and retracted, or inverted, a hole may be cut in the bra the equivalent size of the aerola. (The dark area around the nipple.) This will help make the nipples more prominent. True inverted nipples are rare and the best treatment is to wear Woolwich Shields in the last weeks of pregnancy and, possibly, between feeds after the baby is born. Flat nipples are much more common and usually unfold with stimulation.

6. Taking a good vitamin supplement during pregnancy especially Vitamin A & D may increase resistance to chafing and tenderness of the nipple.

7. The GP or the Practice Nurse can encourage the woman (and her husband) to share thoughts and ideas.

8. Help the woman (and the husband) to talk over with hospital staff the needs of a nursing mother. ? Rooming in from birth and demand feeding and no supplements of water or milk mixture.

– From La Leche League Literature

Figure 7   Breast care during pregnancy

E17

The Management of the Patient on Chemical Contraceptives

Initial

1. Well woman questionnaire and examination (Section C)

Enquire particularly about: migraine, irregular bleeding or discharge. F.H. hypertension. jaundice, history of toxaemia of pregnancy, thrombophlebitis, deep vein thrombosis pulmonary embolism or depression

Include SGOT in biochemical screen

Follow-Up 2 months and 6 monthly thereafter

1. ? any problems

2. Weight

3. B.P.

4. Breast and pelvic examination in older women

5. Endocervical swab. Stuart medium.
6. Cervical smear every two years

7. ? offer rubella vaccine if previous rubella titre negative

1. Scrutinise staff records

2. Choose agent

(a) First choice oestrogen/progesterone combination with an oestrogen content not greater than 50 microgrammes.

(b) Second choice continuous progestogen. (Not reliable as contraceptive for first three days of therapy)

(c) Third choice. In young women having contraception prescribed For the first time and in women who have had side effects from other contraceptives, consider the use of oestrogen/progestogen combination containing oestrogen 30 microgrammes.

3. Prescribe for two months initially

4. Arrange follow up 2 months.

The Morning-After Pill
Must be taken within 72 hours of unprotected intercourse. Stilboestrol mgm 25 enteric-coated b.d. with anti-emetic for 5 days.

Note If the woman taking OC's suffers from gastroenteritis, the compounds may not be absorbed.
Dilantin increases the metabolic rate of oestrogens and there may be a risk of pregnancy with low dosage O.C's.

Contra-indications to oestrogen-containing pill

1. Absolute contra-indications

(a) A history of severe thrombophlebitis, deep vein thrombosis or pulmonary embolism.

(b) Neoplasms of the breast or reproductive organs.

(c) Severe cardiovascular disease.

2. Relative contra-indications

In patients with these complications, individual investigations and follow-up is required. In some it may be possible to continue pill therapy, while in others it may be necessary to use another form of contraception.

(a) Hypertension

(b) Women over the age of 40 years, particularly if they smoke and are overweight, or hypertensive, have diabetes mellitus, hyperlipidaemia or a family history of C.H.D.

(c) Past history of jaundice or liver disease.

(d) Oligomenorrhoea

(e) Low oestrogen – dosage compounds are acceptable where the patient is on insulin and the diabetes well-controlled

After Prof. John Richards
and Dr. Bala Patel

Figure 8   Management of the patient on chemical contraceptives

The Routine Care of the Child At Birth

B2

LOOK FOR:
? Intact and normal-looking with
normal motor tone
? normal facies
? Cataracts
Any deformity neck, arms, legs & digits
Fontanelles
Downs syndrome
Micro ophthalmia
Cleft palate
Diaphragmatic hernia
Cardiac abnormality
Single umbilical artery
? abdominal mass (including renal)
Pilonidal sinus
Spina bifida
Hypospadias
Imperforate anus
Testes
? force of urinary stream
? femoral pulses
C.D.H.
Talipes

HOSPITAL TEST:
Guthrie Test

RECORD:
Familial history
Antenatal history
Apgar rating
Birth weight
Length
Head Circumference ⎤ Record in
⎦ Percentiles

Encourage mother/child contact in the
immediate neonatal period (See Page B23 for
the approach to the Prevention of Emotional
Disorders)

– Recall 10-14 days

APGAR SCALE
Record Score 1 min and 5 mins after
Delivery of Baby

The baby is rated 0, 1 or 2 for each of
the five signs listed in the left-hand
column. The over-all score of 0 to 10
is the sum of the ratings of the five
individual signs. Infants with a score
of 4 or less need help with breathing.

Discuss with a paediatrician:
1. All babies who become clinically
   jaundiced in the first 24 hours
2. Premature infants whose bilirubin
   has reached a level of 10 mg.
3. Full term infants whose bilirubin
   has reached a level of 12 mg.
4. Any jaundiced infant who has, in
   addition, lethargy, anorexia,
   vomiting or pale stools

SIGN	0	1	2
HEART RATE	ABSENT	SLOW (BELOW 100)	OVER 100
RESPIRATORY	ABSENT	SLOW IRREGULAR	GOOD CRYING
MUSCLE TONE	FLACCID	SOME FLEXION OF EXTREMITIES	ACTIVE MOTION
IRRITABILITY REFLEX	NO RESPONSE	GRIMACE	CRY
COLOUR	BLUE, PALE	BODY PINK EXTREMITIES BLUE	COMPLETELY PINK

The indications for active resuscitation (see page E27) are:
a. A baby severely depressed at birth (Heart rate under 100, judged by auscultation, inspection or
   palpatation for a few seconds only) or,
b. A baby not breathing properly at 1 minute after delivery or later

Figure 9   The routine examination at birth

Screening for the Dysmature Infant

No one of these tests is conclusive. The infant's response to all of them is a measure of its maturity

Test 1 Glabellar tap

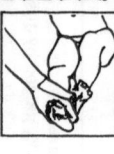

Full term

The infant is tapped lightly over the glabellar region.
Full term Infant – Eyelid muscles contract, but not facial muscles.
Premature Infant – Reflex absent below 32 weeks.
Dysmature Infant – Responds as full term infant.

Test 2 Heel to ear manoeuvre

The hip is flexed so that the thigh is in contact with the abdomen.

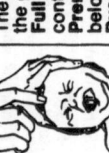

Full term   Premature

Full term Infant – There is difficulty in taking the heel close to the ear and the knee cannot be fully extended (usually about 20° of flexion remains).
Premature Infant – The foot can be taken to the side of the head with toes near the ear and the knee can be fully extended.
Dysmature Infant – Responds as full term infant.

Test 3 Scarf sign

In some infants it is possible to wrap the arm around the neck like a scarf.

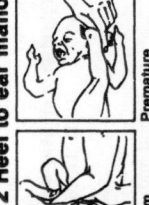

Full term   Premature

Full term Infant – There is marked resistance to the manoeuvre with the elbow barely passing the mid-line.
Premature Infant – Little or no resistance with the manoeuvre with the elbow passing well beyond the mid-line.
Dysmature Infant – Responds as full term infant.

Test 4 Wrist and ankle flexion

The hand or foot is flexed at the wrist or ankle.

Full term   Premature

Full term Infant – Flexion is complete with the hand or foot making contact with arm or shin respectively.
Premature Infant – Only partial flexion can be achieved. A space or 'window' remains between hand and forearm or foot and shin.
Dysmature Infant – Responds as full term infant.

Test 5 Head rotation

The head is gently rotated.

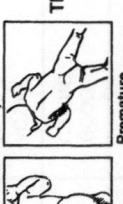

Full term   Premature

Full term Infant – Rotation is possible until the chin is in line with the acromion. Further rotation is impossible without force.
Premature Infant – Rotation is achieved without resistance and the chin passes the acromion.
Dysmature Infant – Responds as full term infant.

Test 6 Plantar creases

Full term   Premature

Full term Infant – the sole is completely smooth and creaseless.
Premature Infant – The sole is covered with creases.
Dysmature Infant – Appears as full term infant.

Test 7 Crossed extensor reflex

Baby supine, one leg extended, foot stimulated.
Full term Infant – The opposite leg flexes at the hip and knee, followed by extension of both hip and knee accompanied by adduction towards the noxious stimulus and fanning of the toes.
Premature Infant – Flexion and extension at the hip and knee are unco-ordinated with little adduction or fanning of the toes.
Dysmature Infant – Responds as full term infant.

Test 8 Posture

The baby is prone

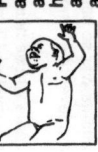

Full term   Premature

Full term Infant – The buttocks are held high with the knees together beneath the abdomen.
Premature Infant – Lies flat with chest and abdomen in contact with surface. Buttocks are low, hips abducted and knees spread wide apart.
Dysmature Infant – Appears as full term infant.

Test 9 Moro reflex

Baby supine. The head is raised one inch and allowed to drop.
Full term Infant – The infant appears startled and throws its arms away from the body. The hands open as the arms are abducted; then the arms are adducted across the chest as if in an embrace.
Premature Infant – The response is incomplete with abduction but little or no adduction.
Dysmature Infant – Responds as full term infant.

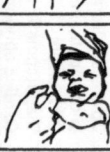

Full term

– Adapted with permission John Wyeth & Bro. (N.Z.) Ltd. (Scripted Dr P.N. Halliday)

Figure 10   Screening for the dysmature infant

The Routine Care of the Child

After Discharge From Hospital Age About Two Weeks

General assessment.

Special attention where there is history of obstetric difficulties or familial congenital abnormalities.

Fontanelles

? Cyanosis or cardiac murmur

? C.D.H.

Check Practice Staff records

? any problems

Length
Weight
Head circumference } Record in Percentiles

Birthmarks

Assess general development and milestones

Test for phenylketonuria and other inborn errors of metabolism (Guthrie card)

Arrange for delivery and labour record to be included in infant's records

Check fluoride administration to mother or child

Encourage breast feeding

– This is the time when some mothers, particularly if inexperienced, are feeling timorous and inadequate. Encouragement, support and goodwill are most helpful

– Recall age 6 weeks

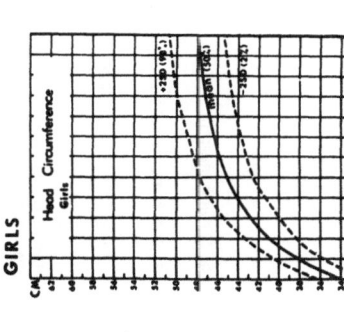

The Auckland Hospital Charts – by courtesy Dr J. Dilworth Matthews.

Figure 11   The routine examination at 2 weeks of age

B3

The Routine Care of the Child

6 weeks of age (mother's postnatal)

Note: The achievement of milestones depends upon development. The apparent delay in an immature infant can lead to unnecessary anxiety.

MILESTONES
Check with mother or examine

GROSS MOTOR
Ventral suspension – head held up momentarily in same plane as rest of body. Some extension of hips and flexion of knees. Flexion of elbows

Prone – pelvis high, but knees no longer under abdomen. Much intermittent extension of hips. Chin raised intermittently off couch. Head turned to one side

Pull to sit – head lag considerable but not complete

Held in sitting position – intermittently hold head up

Held standing – no walking reflex. Head sags forward

May hold head up momentarily

HANDS
Often open. Grasp reflex may be lost

GENERAL UNDERSTANDING
Smiles at mother in response to overtures

VISION
Eyes fixate on objects. They follow moving persons. In supine – looks at object held in midline, following it as it moves from the side to midline. (90 degrees)

General assessment   Length

Fontanelles   Weight   Record in Percentiles

? Evidence brain damage   Head circumference

? Cyanosis or cardiac murmur

Palpate radial and femoral pulses   ? Strabismus (light source)

? C.D.H. limbs movement & function   Birthmarks

Iron administration to premature infants multiple births and those known to have neonatal haemorrhage.   Assess general development and milestones

Encourage fluoride administration

? any problems   Recall age 3 months

The main purpose of the examination at 6 weeks is to check the three H's:
- Head
- Heart
- Hips

See Page B24 for the approach to Preventive Emotional Care

B4

Figure 12   The routine examination at 6 weeks of age

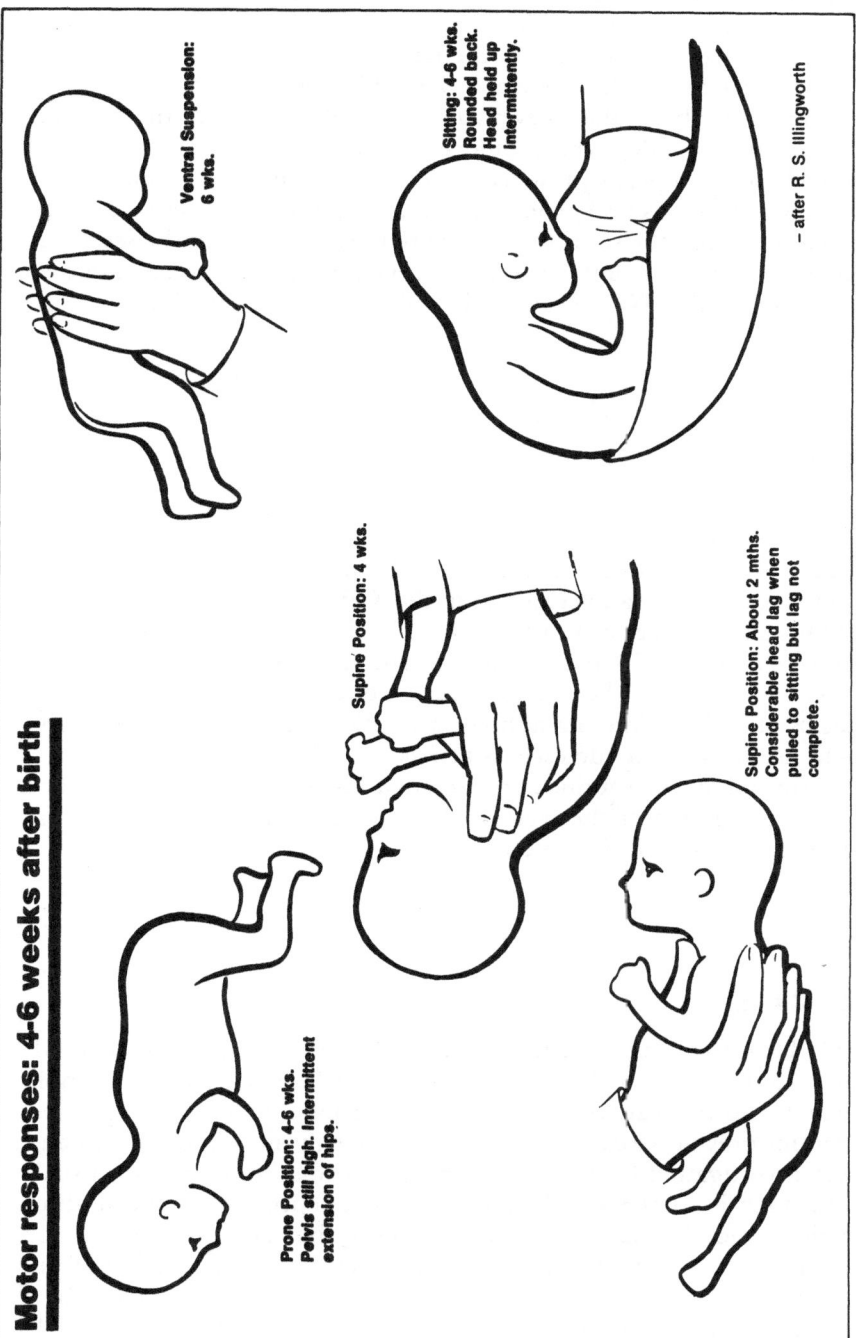

Motor responses: 4-6 weeks after birth

Ventral Suspension: 6 wks.

Sitting: 4-6 wks. Rounded back. Head held up intermittently.

– after R. S. Illingworth

Supine Position: 4 wks.

Prone Position: 4-6 wks. Pelvis still high. Intermittent extension of hips.

Supine Position: About 2 mths. Considerable head lag when pulled to sitting but lag not complete.

Figure 13   Motor responses 4-6 weeks after birth

logy. It is possible for the GP, either in group/or solo practice, to deliver a routine preventive service to infants and school children if he works with the practice nurse. The benefits to the patient can be great. Much of the routine work is done by the nurse and the GP is available when needed. It is convenient to base the surveillance of children upon the routine immunization schedule, which differs in each country. The protocols should include appropriate growth and development charts and milestones of development for easy reference. A simple recall or reminder system for the parent increases the rate of immunization. Guidelines can be set down for both emergency care and for routine preventive health care. Samples of the protocols used in New Zealand for child care are to be found on pp. 105–11.

ADOLESCENT CARE

Adolescents respond well to someone who is willing to listen and who expresses interest by asking concerned questions. Nowhere is it more important to maintain confidentiality. If the parents wish to know what goes on between the adolescent and the GP, the doctor must say 'I understand that you are concerned but you will understand how necessary it is that I should not discuss one person with another. You must trust me to act as I think best'. The practice social worker should be familiar with the basics of family planning and contraception and be supported if she needs to use these with adolescents at risk.

The protocol for the routine approach to a 14-year old is shown on page 111. As usual, much of the work is done by the practice nurse but the doctor is available (see Figure 20).

ADULT CARE

Sensible health care is what is needed in the local community. The GP should be able to deal with common problems (this does not mean simple problems), and be available for the relief of distress, and for emergencies. Any routine preventive care should take cost-effectiveness into account and the over-investigation for rare disorders is to be discouraged. As is usual, the kind of service that is supplied to the patient depends upon the needs of the patient and the particular circumstances, but simple protocols for routine adult preventive health care can be set down. Also, much of the approach to emergency care can be systematized. A simple protocol for a routine examination of the adult woman is included in Figure 21. Investigations are few and, again, the practice staff does a lot of the routine work, leaving the doctor to listen and be available.

B1

Routine Preventive Care in the First 14 Years of Life

AGE	DOCTOR	PRACTICE STAFF	PRESENT SCHEDULE OF CHILDHOOD IMMUNISATION
Birth	X		
2 weeks	X	X	
6 weeks	X	X	
3 months		X	Trivac. Polio
5 months		X	Trivac. Polio
9 months		X	
1 year	X	X	Morbilli
18 months		X	Dip-Tet. Polio
3 years		X	
5 years	X	X	Dip-Tet. Rubella
7 years		X	
10 years	X	X	Tetanus
14 years	X	X	

Consultation Plan

Those consultations marked with an asterisk include suggestions about the kind of interview advocated by Dr Kevin Cullen of Australia and are designed to help in the prevention of emotional disorders in pre-school children.

The interview at 9 months is the time when the Health Dept would like all infants to be examined by the GP. There seems to be no special reason why this particular age was chosen but it fits in well with Dr. Cullen's approach.

The protocols for the Prevention of Emotional Disorders in Pre-School Children are placed at the end of Section B following the percentile anthropomorphic charts (on pages B23-B30).

Figure 14 Consultation plan

B9

The Routine Care of the Child

18 months of age

Length — Record in
Weight — Percentiles
Head circumference

Assess general development and
milestones ? problems

Teeth

Refer Doctor if necessary

Check fluoride administration

Polio vaccine

Dip - Tet vaccine

Arrange haemoglobin estimation.

Discuss with Mother:
Use of seat belts.
Barriers around pools and against street traffic.
Precautions in home against:
Boiling fluids
Matches and fires
Sharp instruments and
dangerous toys
Drugs, household poisons particularly
weedicides and herbicides

Encourage both parents to read and tell stories

Recall Age 3 years.

MILESTONES
Check with mother or examine

GROSS MOTOR
Gets up and down stairs, holding rail, without help
Walks up stairs, one hand held
Walks, pulling toy or carrying doll
Seats self on chair.
Beginning to jump (both feet).

CUBES
Tower of 3 or 4

BALL
Throws ball without fall

DRESSING
Takes off gloves, socks, unzips

FEEDING
Manages spoon well, without rotation

PENCIL
Spontaneous scribble Makes stroke imitatively

GENERAL UNDERSTANDING
"Domestic mimicry". Copies mother in dusting,
washing, cleaning

PARTS OF BODY
Points to 2 or 3 (nose, eye, hair etc.)

PICTURE CARD
Points to one ("Where is the . . .?")

BOOK
Turns pages, 2 or 3 at a time.
Points to picture of car or dog.
Shows sustained interest

SPHINCTER CONTROL Dry by day; occasional accident

SPEECH: Jargon. Many intelligible words

SIMPLE FORMBOARD Piles 3 blocks

Figure 15   The routine examination at 18 months of age

The Routine Care of the Child

5 years of age – pre school

General assessment:

Eyes

Ears

Nose

Mouth and teeth

Throat

C.V.S. – Pulses radial and femoral

R.S.

A.S. ? hernia

Testes

Limbs

Check Practice Staff records

? problems

Height ⎤
Weight ⎦ Record in Percentiles

B.P.

Assess general development and milestones

Visual acuity – E card

Hearing – audiometry (6 frequencies)

Arrange urinalysis

Check fluoride administration

Mention importance of nutritional school lunches

Dip – Tet vaccine and Rubella vaccine

Recall Age 7 Years

Diagnosis of short stature due to isolated growth hormone deficiency should be possible by the age of 5

MILESTONES
Check with mother or examine

GROSS MOTOR
Skips on both feet

PENCIL
Copies triangle

GENERAL UNDERSTANDING
Gives age

Distinguishes morning from afternoon

Compares 2 weights

COLOURS
Names 4

PREPOSITION (Triple order)
'Put this on the chair,
open the door,
then give me that book'

B11

Figure 16   The routine examination at 5 years of age

The Routine Care of the Child

The Child New to the Practice Questionnaire

Any information set down here will be confidential to the Doctors records.

Surname:	Address:		Parents occupation:	Date of Entry	Date of Birth:	Account No.
			Solo parent ☐ NO ☐			
Forename:		Telephone:	Widowed ☐ Separated ☐			

YES ☐ NO ☐

A. Are there any brothers or sisters?
   If so, state sex and ages ....
   ....

B. Was the pregnancy and birth abnormal or unusual? ☐
   If so, what was abnormal? ....
   ....

C. Do you think the child has not developed normally? ☐
   If so, how is the child not normal? ....
   ....
   At what age did the child walk? ....
   At what age did the child talk? ....
   At what age did the child achieve bladder control,
   by day? .... And at night? ....

D. Does the child go to school? If so, ☐

E. Are you dissatisfied or unhappy with the school achievement? ☐

F. Has the child missed any routine immunisations?
   Could you list what immunisations the child has had? (with dates)
   ....
   ....

G. Has the child any allergies? ☐
   If so, what are they? ....
   ....

YES ☐ NO ☐

H. Is there any history of illness? ☐ ☐
   If so, what were the illnesses? (Give age) ....
   ....

I. Are there any previous medical records? ☐ ☐
   If so, where are they? ....

J. Has the child any other physical complaints? ☐ ☐
   If so, what are they? ....
   ....

K. Has the child any emotional problem you would
   like to discuss with Doctor? ☐ ☐

L. Is there any family history of illnesses? ☐ ☐
   If so, what are they? ....

M. Can you think of any other way the child may
   need help? ☐ ☐
   If so, what would you suggest? ....
   ....

B15

Figure 17   The child new to the practice questionnaire

Paediatric Emergencies

Convulsions:

1. When the call for help arrives advise parent to
   (a) Place the child on its side. This is usually enough to keep the airway clear.
   (b) Refrain from attempts to control any convulsive movements
   (c) Protect the tongue from being bitten
   (d) If there is a pyrexia, tepid-sponge the child

2. Try to see the patient within 5 minutes

3. If the convulsion is still in progress, administer at once intravenous valium 2.5 mg (some risk) or intramuscular sod. phenobarb 6 mg – kg. stat.

4. If the child is still convulsing 10 minutes after the injection, repeat the dose.

5. If after another 5 minutes the child is still convulsing, consider hospital admission.

6. Exclude meningitis. If in doubt, arrange lumbar puncture.

7. If the criteria for a true benign febrile convulsion are not present, consider the diagnosis further.

   The criteria are:
   (a) Fever of 39°C or more
   (b) Age between 6 months and 3 years
   (c) Family history of B.F.C.
   (d) No clinical evidence of C.N.S. pathology
   (e) Duration less than 10 minutes
   (f) Any E.E.G. should be normal

8. If the patient is less than 6 months of age, arrange hospital admission for organic disease is more likely.

9. Over the age of 4 years the cause is likely to be epilepsy and the treatment should be administered at home.

Poisons:

1. Reach the child or have it brought in as soon as pos-. poison. Instruct parent to bring the container to the surge.

2. Except where there is ingestion of caustics or hydrocarbons the stomach should be emptied as soon as possible. Emesis is more effective than lavage. Administer a single dose of syrup of ipecacuanha

3. If vomiting does not result within 15 minutes, the same dose may be repeated while arrangements are made gastric lavage to be carried out if emesis still fails to occur

4. If the poison is an acid, dilute the acid (or instruct the parent to dilute the acid) with water or milk or milk of magnesia. Do not induce emesis

5. If the poison is an alkali use copious fluids to dilute (or instruct the patient to use dilute vinegar or lemon juice.) Do not induce emesis

6. Observation and cardiorespiratory monitoring (beware tricyclic antidepressants) may be necessary

After Prof. J.M. Watt

Dose of Syrup of Ipecac

Children 1 year 15 ml 200 ml orange juice
        2 years 20 ml
        3 years 25 ml
        over 3 years 30 ml
Adults 50 ml

The Most Dangerous Drugs
1. Tricyclic antidepressants
2. Aminophylline
3. Paracetamol
4. Glutithemide (doriden)

E3

Figure 18   Paediatric emergencies – poisoning and convulsions

The Management of Gastroenteritis In Infancy

Gastroenteritis is common under the age of 2 years and is seen rarely in fully breast-fed infants. It is usually a temporary upset and seems to often accompany the acquisition of new strains of coliforms.

Virus infection is responsible for more than 50 per cent of cases but bacterial infection, administration of drugs, surgical problems (intussusception) and giardia infection can produce diarrhoea.

Signs of Dehydration
Are Those of Renal Insufficiency:

1. Dry naps
2. Skin turgor
3. Depressed fontanelle
4. Dry lips and sticky tongue
5. Acetone on the breath
6. Loss of muscle tone
7. Lethargy
8. Tachycardia

Diagnosis and assessment:

1. Are the symptoms and signs compatible with gastroenteritis? Watch for intestinal obstruction, pyloric stenosis or intussusception

2. Are there signs of infection in other systems to which the diarrhoea and vomiting may be secondary?

3. Is there any degree of dehydration present? More rapid dehydration may occur in very young babies.

4. Is the mother capable of carrying out treatment? Should the child be admitted to hospital, the doctor or the practice nurse see the child again?

Management:

1. Weigh the child at first and subsequent examinations.

2. Fluid administration in small amounts and frequently is the most important treatment. In mild cases more dilute milk feeds may be used. In more severe cases withdraw all milk and solid feeds, and replace by suitable salt containing clear fluid such as "Isolyte O" or "Lytren" which are better prepared by the pharmacist. Under the age of 6 months use "Isolyte O" as "Lytren" can make the diarrhoea worse (Dissacharride intolerance or overdose).

3. Do not use thickened feeds, unrestricted glucose solutions, antidiarrhoeal preparations antiemetics or antibiotics or any other drugs.

4. Feeds should not be more than 100 ml and should be administered every one or two hours initially. After 48 hours a return can be made to dilute milk feeds and normal feeding may be possible within a week. If there is no improvement in 48 hours, consider admission to hospital.

5. Admission to hospital is indicated when the signs of dehydration are present or the condition of the child has deteriorated with treatment.

– After Dr Terry Casely
and Mary Hay R.N.

E4

Figure 19   Gastroenteritis in infancy

The Routine Care of the Child

14 years of age

B14

General Assessment	Testes	
Eyes	Limbs	
Ears		
Nose	? Problems	
Mouth and teeth		
Throat		
C.N.S.		
Breasts		
R.S.		
A.S.		

Practice Staff

Height ⎤
Weight ⎦ Record in Percentiles

Blood pressure

Visual acuity – distance type

Hearing – audiometry (6 frequencies)

Record date menarche and menstrual history in girls

? Smoker

? School progress

Arrange – urinalysis
       – mass chest X-Ray
       – Heaf test

Girls – administer booster rubella vaccine

Figure 20   The routine examination at 14 years of age

The Adult Woman Examination

EXAMINE: Skin

Hair

Eyes

Face

Mouth

Throat

Thyroid

Breasts

Heart

Lungs

Abdomen

Hernial orifices

Pelvis

Rectum

Limbs

Nails

TAKE: Cervical smear

Cervical swab

? Any problems

? contraception

Questionnaire. Start basic data and record flow chart.

Weight – clothed. Height

Prepare for examination

Temperature

Blood pressure

Provide cervical smear tray (label slide)

Provide swab and Stuart medium (label)

On cervical smear requisition form note:
– Age
– LMP
– If there is history of cervical surgery

ARRANGE: – Mass miniature chest film

– P.C.V.

– Serum cholesterol and triglycerides

– 2 hrs. p.c. Blood sugar

– Urinalysis

RECALL: Case notes and reports

investigations to be assessed 14 days.

Figure 21   The adult woman examination

The Elderly Woman or Man Examination

C6

EXAMINE:

Skin

Hair

Eyes ?V.A.

Ears ?Audiometry

Face

Mouth

Throat

Thyroid

Breasts

Heart

Lungs

Abdomen

Hernial orifices

Pelvis

Rectum

Limbs, including feet

Nails

Woman: Cervical smear
cervical swab

Man: prostate
scrotum & testes

? any problems

Questionnaire. Start basic data and record flow chart

Weight (clothed). Height

Prepare for examination

Temperature

Blood pressure, lying and standing

Ocular tensions where there is FH of glaucoma

Woman: Provide cervical smear tray (label slide, name, age)
Provide swab and stuart medium (label name, age, vag)
On cervical smear requisition form note age and if there is a
history of cervical surgery

ARRANGE: – F.S. Chest film
– Full blood screen
– Serum creatinine
– 2 hr p.c. blood sugar
– Arthritis screen
– Estimation of thyroid function
– Serum electrolytes
– Urinalysis, microscopy & culture

– After Dr B. B. Taylor

Figure 22   The routine examination of the elderly woman or man

The adult woman routine examination (see Figure 21)

THE ELDERLY PATIENT

Care of elderly people is best carried out in the local community. The role of centralized, specialized services is to back up the GP and the local team. Voluntary effort and local self-help is to be encouraged, as is community participation in the care of the elderly. The training of the practice nurse will be extended, inevitably, to include the basics of social work with elderly people, and the GP must be familiar with the principles. Both must understand the range of services available to the patient and be willing to use them.

Interpersonal problems may be just as acute and as important as with any younger person and just as amenable to the listening ear and interested help. There is an excellent practical textbook on geriatric care by Anderson (Anderson, 1976), and a simple protocol for the routine examination of the elderly patient is shown in Figure 22.

HIGH-INCIDENCE CHRONIC ILLNESS

Preventive and maintenance care in high-incidence chronic illness is a task that falls within the services provided by the GP. The expansion of medical technology has been great and the practice nurse can often deliver it more efficiently than the GP, particularly if she has his support and backing. As usual, the mere routine management of illness does not constitute proper medical care; there is still the task of helping the patient. The care of chronic illness can often be systematized.

TERMINAL CARE AND THE DYING PATIENT

It is said that to be comfortable with the dying patient one must have accepted one's own inevitable death. Be that as it may, the comfort of an interested doctor who has known the patient and the family can relieve a great deal of distress. Also, the preventive health opportunities are just as great in the bereavement situation as anywhere else. Doctors always feel they could have done more when a patient dies.

Visit relatives of the deceased as soon as possible, and keep in touch for the ensuing weeks and even up to 12 months, for it is a vulnerable time for the bereaved. Practice nurses and the practice social worker can do this too. If a patient should die, say in hospital, and the information is delayed, the relatives should be visited as soon as is possible.

The anatomy and the pathology of grief have been defined and any health professional should understand the feelings and be able to help. The person who is dying and the relatives have the same kind of feelings and the final stage is acceptance of separation and loss.

The dying are lonely. The prospect of dying is painful to the patient, the relatives and the health professionals. Often we treat a dying patient with

Management of Diabetes Mellitus

1. Diagnosis begins with glycosuria or raised blood sugar. Accept blood sugar over 11.1 mmol/L (200 mg dL), otherwise G.T.T.
2. Physical examination including fundi for micro-aneurysms and peripheral circulation. Record blood sugars, weight, height, B.P. Define ideal weight.
3. Start patient education–nature of diabetes, long term complications, importance of ideal weight, diet, exercise, stop smoking, monitoring of blood sugars, restoration of health energy, minimal interference with life style, care of the feet.
4. Possible trial period without drugs or insulin with monitoring of blood sugars and frequent follow-up. Invoke expertise of dietician (with partner). CHO (unrefined) should be above 40% total calories; reduce fat to 30% total calories.
5. Select an antidiabetic agent if necessary.
6. Keep up education and re-stress importance of recording.
7. If insulin is used decide on initial dose. Instruct in use of insulin and technique. Daily supervision.
8. Regular follow-up. Continue education. Decide on insulin or drug dosage. Continue monitoring and recording. Ultimate aim is for patient to take over control with the personal doctor as backup.

No matter how much education is delivered in the initial stages, the education needs to be repeated and continued over the years.

Insulin Therapy:

The idea is to replace insulin in the right amounts at the right time.

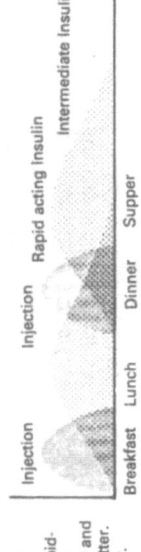

Normal Insulin Reponse

Breakfast   Lunch   Dinner   Supper

– a single injection of an intermediate insulin in the morning seldom works. There is not enough insulin for breakfast or dinner and too much between meals.

Injection   Intermediate Insulin

Breakfast   Lunch   Dinner   Supper

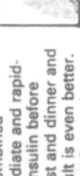
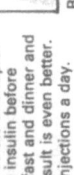

– add a rapid-acting insulin to the morning intermediate insulin and another dose of rapid-acting before dinner. This is better but here is not enough insulin during the night. Two injections a day.

Injection   Injection   Rapid acting Insulin   Intermediate Insulin

Breakfast   Lunch   Dinner   Supper

– use combined intermediate and rapid-acting insulin before breakfast and dinner and the result is even better. Two injections a day.

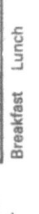
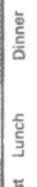
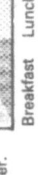
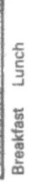

Injection   Injection   Rapid acting insulin   Intermediate Insulin

Breakfast   Lunch   Dinner   Supper

– but to get best results use rapid-acting insulin before each main meal. Add intermediate insulin to the injection before dinner. Three injections a day.

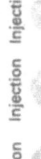

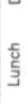
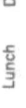
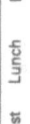
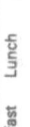
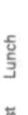

Injection   Injection   Injection   Rapid acting Insulin   Intermediate Insulin

Breakfast   Lunch   Dinner   Supper

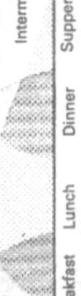
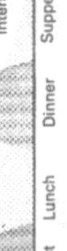
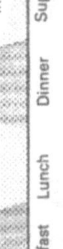

Figure 23   The management of diabetes mellitus

The Management of Hypertension

1. **Confirm the hypertension**
Readings are taken on three different occasions.

Initial investigations can include:
-C.B.C.
-fasting blood sugar
-fasting lipids
-urinalysis

2. **Examination**
(? cause for the hypertension, coincidental disease, organ damage).

Additional investigations can be:
-serum electrolytes
-creatinine
-uric acid
-E.C.G.
-I.V.P. (if there is evidence of renal involvement)
-creatinine clearance

Special attention:
-smoking or alcohol abuse
-any drugs taken which could raise the BP (chemical contraceptives, vasoconstrictors, analgesics carbenoxolone and liquorice analogues)
-whether a great deal of salt is consumed
-is patient taking enough exercise?
-whether there is any psychological stress

at home or at work
-is the patient overweight?
-what is the expiratory peak flow? (use the Mini-Wright)
-are there palpable femoral pulses on both sides, weak, or delayed in relation to the radial pulse
-is there a carotid bruit, abdominal or femoral bruit?
-do the retinae show significant abnormalities?
-is there hyperlipidaemia or diabetes?

3. **Start education**

4. **Is the drug treatment necessary?**
It may be enough to change the lifestyle (reduce weight, stop smoking, reduce salt and alcohol intake and consider the psychological pressures).

5. **If drugs are considered necessary:**
-*are any hypotensive agents contraindicated?*
-*how does the patient feel about being hypertensive* and the need to take drugs? Does the patient understand the need for probable life-long routine medication and is the patient willing to cooperate?
-*select the antihypertensive agent.* Younger patients with mild hypertension may do well on a beta blocker alone. A beta blocker is more specifically indicated with angina, sinus tachycardia, frequent ectopics or migraine. A diuretic should be

included specifically with poor myocardial reserve, dyspnoea and fluid retention.
-*the drug regime should be as simple as possible* and the initial dose, small.

6. **If possible, instruct patient how to monitor own BP at home.**

7. **Arrange weekly appointments** until the BP is controlled and stable, the patient is comfortable and compliance is established. Keep up education.

8. **Follow up in one month and after that three monthly and record BP, weight and** assess compliance (patients bring tablet containers to the consultation) and comfort. Communicate with non-attenders.

9. **Annual Checkup**
Assess:
-Patient's point of view, record of home compliance
-control of BP and weight
-evidence of organ damage
-any side effects from the drugs.

At annual checkup investigations can include:
-C.B.C.
-urinalysis
-serum creatinine
-electrolytes
-uric acid
-expiratory peak flow

Figure 24   The management of hypertension

lies, half-truths and conspiracies of silence, and the result is that the patient is poignantly lonely. It is so easy to fall back on treating only the physical disease.

Doctors and nurses are afraid of the dying. Ours is a death-denying society. We tend to die in hospitals rather than at home. Doctors are on the side of health and feel failures with death. Yet the mortality of life is 100 per cent. The dying patient may not communicate clearly because it may make the health professional and relatives uncomfortable.

Often there is a conspiracy situation – a charade. There may be an unspoken pact by patients, doctors and relatives not to talk of the terminal nature of the illness – 'I know the nature of the illness but I will not believe it'. The doctor should not allow himself to participate in the conspiracy situation. If the relatives request the patient must not be told, the doctor should reply 'I understand what you say but you must leave it to me to do the right thing as I see it'.

What does the dying patient want? To know that someone cares, understands, and will help the patient come to terms with himself, his illness and his family, and relieve his distress and discomfort.

Should the patient be told? Most dying patients know what is happening and it is often a great relief to be able to speak about it. The patient must always be given the truth as he or she asks for it. The doctor may choose not to tell all, but he always listens. The question 'Am I going to die?' can always be answered with the kind of question that is gentle and opens up further areas of feeling such as 'How would you feel about that?' The most valuable asset is a pre-existing good relationship between patient and doctor. If it is possible to talk about impending death, anxiety often diminishes.

Not all patients want to know. Some, although aware of impending death choose to ignore the reality. It is possible to make a will, give away possessions and make farewells yet behave as though life will go on. This is the person's privilege.

There are **five stages in the feelings of the dying and the bereaved:**

Stage I: *Denial.* The patient or the bereaved relative has a feeling of unreality, 'as though it is not happening'.

Stage II: *Feeling returns.* The loss is beginning to be felt and there is resentment about this. The patient or relative is not angry against the doctor or nurse but is saying 'Why me?' It is necessary to accept the anger and resentment.

Stage III: *Bargaining.* With God or the attendants to carry on a bit longer. The nurse and the doctor understand this but do not enter into the process.

Stage IV: *Depression.* This is profound and normal. It is deep mourning and a feeling of the loss, the separation. The nurse and the doctor can mourn with the patient often without saying very much.

Stage V: *Acceptance.* The ultimate goal.

The dying child: This is the most painful of all. The plea for compassion and honesty in relationships extends to the dying child who knows early on how his parents feel. It is not necessary to go on plying the child with uncomfortable treatments after the battle is clearly lost.

The family must be helped too. The relatives need help before and after the bereavement. There is no side-stepping the process of grief which must be carried to completion. The relatives must be involved at every point and unfounded fears (for example, that cancer is contagious or familial) must be dealt with. It is important to understand that there is often not much immediate satisfaction in helping the bereaved. The health professional cannot give back the lost life.

Cot deaths. Patients go through the same sequence but with the added weight of guilt that they were, possibly, in some way responsible for the death. Here, above all, it is important to have a pre-existing doctor–patient relationship. Communication with others who have experienced sudden infant death can help.

The relief of physical distress. Pain and physical distress is often less when mental distress is reduced and much pain can be relieved without resorting to analgesics. It is important to listen to the patient and identify the facets of distress. Relief of constipation, adequate hydration, antibiotics, physiotherapy and oxygen may be useful. Analgesics range from aspirin variants to morphine which should be given by mouth if possible. Non-steroidal anti-inflammatory agents may help with the pain of bone secondaries. There is no room for 'meddlesome medicine' and no need to prolong life unnecessarily (Kubler-Ross, 1970).

COUNSELLING OR PSYCHOTHERAPY

The basics of counselling are simple. The practice nurse, who has great opportunities for preventive work, should be familiar with the techniques as well as the GP and the practice social worker.

*The therapist must care what happens to the patient.
*The therapist must be able to listen to the expression of the patient's feelings with all the senses and be able to tolerate what is said.
*The ability to establish a good relationship early on is important.
*Confidentiality is essential. Record in the practice records only what is approved of by the patient.
*Therapy should be non-authoritarian and non-directive as far as is possible.
*The technique is to help the patient to explore his/her own situation, express hostility and hurt feelings, and identify the basic problem. It is not for the therapist to tell the patient what to do or try to promote a happy ending. If there is a problem, it may be necessary for the patient to identify it, accept that there may not be a magic answer, and work for a solution.

*The message to the patient is that he is able to solve his own problems and help himself, that the psychotherapy is intended to be brief and a help towards this end. The advantages of long-term therapy may not be as great as its hazards which can include the development of a strong transference situation and the mobilization of infantile needs that neither the therapist nor patient can meet.

*The use of tranquillisers should be brief and for the relief of emotional pain while the patient expresses his feelings about a crisis situation.

*The gentle, broad, non-judgemental, probing question is useful as an interview device. Such questions must be accepting, permissive and aid conversation. Examples are: 'That's interesting!', 'What else would you say about that?', 'How do you understand the situation?', 'Why do you think this is so?' and 'How is it you feel this way?'

*If there is a confrontation, it arises out of a concern for the patient and the therapist is willing to be involved. Responsible confrontation is an invitation to self-examination – a caring activity and not an act of punishment. If a patient presents while in therapy with another, find out why this has happened. It may be that the patient is in conflict about his relationship with the other therapist and this may need working out. It may not be in the patient's best interests that you should assume responsibility for therapy at that point.

*The counselling of people whom one knows well socially is very difficult.

*Membership of the therapist in a training-discussion group which meets regularly is most important. Interviews and case histories are reported and discussed and the therapist–patient situation is explored. This is a good way to learn the techniques of counselling.

PRESCRIBING

*The use of drugs should be rational.

*Be conversant with, and use, as small a range of drugs as possible. Use a drug only if it is clearly indicated for the specific condition and the specific patient. In selecting other drugs, be especially alert to their effects, including interactions. When combining drugs, try to avoid using two with similar side-effects.

*Be familiar with the duration of time that the drug exists in the body, particularly tranquillisers.

*Before prescribing, check the patient's record, and ask if he is taking drugs prescribed by another physician. Try to start with one drug or as few as possible. Appreciate that some people are particularly sensitive to drugs.

*Where there is altered physiology or known pathology (especially renal and hepatic) watch for drug reactions.

*Keep a clear record of drug regimens and prescribe as small a quantity as is needed.

*Check for possible sequelae to drug ingestion. The repeating of prescriptions for significant drugs, without supervision, leaves the general practitioner clearly responsible. Also, the continual repeating of prescriptions may conceal an agreement between patient and doctor not to deal with significant problems (Balint, 1970).

References

1. Carson, S. (1975). *A Manual for General Practice*. Auckland, Beecham Research Laboratories.
2. Cullen, K. (1976). *The Prevention of Emotional Disorders in Preschool Children*. Melbourne, Family Medicine Programme, RACGP.
3. Anderson, F. (1976). *Practical Management of the Elderly*. 3rd edition (London: Blackwell Scientific Publications)
4. Kubler-Ross, E. (1969). *On Death and Dying*. (New York: Macmillan)
5. Balint, M. *et al.* (1970). *Treatment or Diagnosis. A Study of Repeat Prescriptions in General Practice*. (London: Tavistock Publications)

7
Patient Education

JOHN FRY (UK) AND ROGER MEYRICK (UK)

FEATURES OF PRIMARY CARE

Because of the special features of primary care, the physician and his team have special opportunities for educating patients on health care and important related matters.

Primary care services have to provide continuing accessible care to the local community. The population cared for is small and relatively static. In developed countries the average population per primary physician tends to be between 2000 and 3000 persons, but is lower in some countries.

Primary care services provide professional first-contact care, but in addition are responsible for long-term and continuing care, extending often over generations and lifetimes of both patients and physicians.

Here then are very special opportunities for patient education because of the very special privileged relationships developed and built up between doctors and patients.

Because the primary physician tends to provide care for relatively small and static populations over many years, he is able to create good professional relations with individuals, families and the community. He is able to become an important figure in the social structure of the local community, relating to many other essential parts of the life of that community including education, housing, town planning, sanitation, transport, nutrition and even politics.

GOOD HEALTH CARE

Good health care requires very much more than the provision of adequate resources in terms of trained physicians, nurses, social workers and the modern physical and technological resources that they will demand and expect.

Medical resources and manpower are not the only factors in attaining and maintaining good health. There are others that are equally, if not more, important.

Good health requires essential basic social and economic conditions so that the people can be adequately fed, housed, educated, employed, occupied, exercised and involved with their living standards.

Good health in the community demands considerable community participation and involvement in preventive, curative and educational health affairs in order to make the best possible use of available resources.

Good health demands a considerable degree of self-reliance and self-help in keeping healthy, in preventing disease, in self-caring for minor ailments, and in collaborating with health professionals in the management of more serious diseases.

WHY PATIENT EDUCATION?

These, therefore, are very strong reasons for seeking individual, family and community collaboration and involvement in health care in its widest sense. Individuals in particular and the public in general tend to be most interested in health matters, and given the encouragement and opportunities will do their best.

Individual, family and public involvement in health matters, however, cannot be left to a general *laissez-faire* exercise where information and guidance are picked up haphazardly through occasional contacts with health professionals, through the public media and other unplanned events.

Patient education, if it is to be effective and successful, has to be planned, has to have objectives, has to have specified content, has to employ special methods, and has to be subject to continuing assessment to measure its results and its effects.

Planning

It is best to have a *plan* when embarking on any hopefully productive action and this is so with patient education. A plan has to have *objectives*, but even before setting these, it is necessary to decide what broad *group* is to be educated.

There is education for the *individual patient* and this may be specific for certain curative or preventive actions, or it may be general, related to a lifestyle that is potentially dangerous to health.

There is education for the *family*. It is well known that in addition to genetic 'soil' factors that may predispose to disease, there also are environmental 'seed' factors. The former are difficult to influence, the latter are amenable to change through changes in behaviour patterns and habits resulting from education and support.

There is education for the *community*. This has been the traditional form of 'health education' through various public media. It is important, but has to be planned well to be effective, with more specific objectives than hitherto.

It is at the local community level that education for better health and self-help can produce very worthwhile results. The primary health team has special opportunities to stimulate, encourage, lead and guide the community in such endeavours.

Objectives

The following are examples of objectives that may be considered for patient education. They are not meant to be comprehensive. Each plan has to set out its own objectives and targets. The more specific, the more practical, and the less ambitious the plan and the targets, the more likely it is to succeed.

A general objective should be to teach a *more honest approach* to the scope and limitations of modern medicine. There has been a tendency to 'oversell' modern medical technological skills and to raise public and professional expectations to unreal and unachievable levels.

There is a need for some 'negative' education on health to emphasize what can be done by whom to improve health, and to emphasize repeatedly the individual's own responsibilities through self-help and by following the simple rules of health – no smoking, less eating, less drinking and more exercise.

It is important to include in any health educational programme the following questions and discussion of their answers.

> *What is 'normal'?* To stress the wide range of normality.
> *What is 'tolerable'?* To stress the inevitable need to accept many common diseases of life.
> *What is 'curable'?* To demonstrate the low rates of actual curability of many disorders, but at the same time to show how their effects can be relieved to make their tolerance possible.
> *What is 'preventable'?* To stress that much prevention is in the individual's, the family's and the community's own hands and that prevention cannot be left to the health services alone.
> *What is 'self-treatable'?* To show how many common conditions can be self-treated without recourse to medical aid.

More specifically further objectives should concentrate on the following:

1. Teaching clearly and honestly the nature, course, outcome, management and prevention of common diseases and problems. This can be done at a personal and individual level during the consultation, or through public education.
2. Compliance and collaboration in following advice given by health professionals.
3. Better self-care. Opportunities often present to show how in future the same problem could be self-treated or even prevented.
4. The use of consultations by primary care workers which offer

excellent opportunities for changing bad personal habits and preventing disease.
5. The early recognition of disease and the significance of important symptoms.
6. The better use of available local health resources and facilities.
7. The promotion of community participation through:
    *assessing local situations
    *defining local problems
    *initiating local action
    *preparing local plans
    *implementing local decisions
    *evaluating local results

SPECIAL AT-RISK GROUPS

In primary care it is possible and important to prepare plans for 'at-risk' groups for whom special education is necessary. These groups have special problems and require specific measures in educating them to help themselves and to collaborate with the health team in their care.
Examples include:
Antenatal care needs a planned programme to prevent problems and to reduce maternal and infant morbidity and mortality.
Child care should be based on a regular programme of planned supervision of the child and education of the mother.
Adolescence presents few major problems to the majority of adolescents, but good patient education and the use of available services may prevent problems and help those who do have problems.
Middle age is the period prior to old age. It is the time when it is too late to prevent some disorders, but it is a time when patient education may alleviate some problems and prevent future problems.
Specific clinical groups should be defined for special patient education and supervision. These include patients with:
*diabetes
*anaemia, and especially pernicious anaemia
*thyroid disorders
*post-operative organ removals – gastrectomy, adrenalectomy, nephrectomy, and so on
*cancer
*obesity
*coronary artery disease
*hypertension
*strokes
*and those on potentially dangerous drugs.

PATIENT EDUCATION DURING THE CONSULTATION

Although most doctors will claim that they undertake health education in every surgery, it is surprising how many consultations, when examined in detail, fail to reveal any significant amount of information other than the statement that the patient should undertake a certain course of treatment, or has a certain disease which may be altered by a particular approach. In spite of this it is well established that the *one-to-one confrontation* which most doctors practise throughout their professional lives is the most effective basis for patient education. It is probable that the patient is more receptive when suffering or anxious because this gives him a motive for learning, and also the doctor a chance to teach. Despite this, few patients remember much of what they are told, (Hugh-Jones *et al.* 1964). Research has shown that things said at the beginning of an interview, in a friendly rather than a brusque or authoritarian way, are remembered best (Francis *et al.* 1969). It is said that in a discussion of the patient's habits, a moderate degree of anxiety and some direct involvement in the consultation is also a help.

Increased difficulty is experienced by those in the older age groups, particularly those over 65, and also by those of a different cultural background from that of the doctor. For all patients, but in particular for these groups, a diagram or a model to assist the explanation, with a pamphlet to take away and read, is helpful.

GROUP DISCUSSION

The recognition of groups at particular risk is referred to earlier in the chapter, and where this has been done, the assembly of groups for health education has been tried. *Small group discussions* appear to be good, if sometimes slow, in changing attitudes. Where a number of people with a similar disability, disease or problem can be brought together in groups of six to ten, the ensuing discussion will quickly allow the alert group organizer an opportunity to introduce new ideas. Patients with obesity, a smoking problem or alcoholism may respond well in this setting (Pommerlan *et al.*, 1975).

Much more difficult is the disparate group, called together to discuss such subjects as retirement preparation or home safety. Here the benefit would seem to be greater by calling together *larger groups* of twenty, thirty, or even fifty. Discussion is usually opened by a leader, and slides and diagrams may be shown. The use of an audiotape from specialist libraries overcomes the problem of finding a knowledgeable speaker. The group leader need not agree with what is said, and it may even help discussion if he can say why, and in what way, his views are different.

POSTERS

Perhaps the longest standing and certainly the most abused approach is that of displaying posters. In spite of this it remains popular, for at least one reason. It works. Their value lies in drawing attention to a subject, and by their very presence they are repetitive. Not all posters are good and many are quite unsuitable for use in medical centres.

When selecting a poster, first consider the impact of that poster on yourself. Is the general design good? Is the layout clear and do the colours attract you? Then examine the printing. The smallest print must be easily readable at the longest distance from which it is likely to be seen. The subject matter must be clear and there must be only one subject dealt with. Now consider where it is to be placed. Will the colours clash with the surroundings? There is a difference between clashing and standing out clearly, and if you do decide to be garish, remember that many sick patients will have to view it at close quarters. Taste is important. Posters will often reflect the type of surgery or the type of doctor that you are. Whilst it may be of primary importance to tackle the problems of venereal disease, sexual perversion and family planning, the majority of younger and older people will be offended if these problems are not approached with care, or if posters are displayed in an inappropriate place.

In some limited circumstances, there are accepted sites for the display of posters of a special kind. These posters contain information of greater detail, such as the address of the Social Welfare Department, the site of an emergency unit, or the names of local organizations which may offer help. If these are to be displayed, they should be kept in one place all the time and quite separate from posters of other types and for other purposes. A number of attempts to extend the effectiveness of posters by the use of spotlights, mobiles hung over them, or different printing effects, have probably done little to enhance their value. With the possible exception of machines which actually change the posters at set intervals of something between ten seconds and two minutes, it is better to stick to a good, well designed sheet (Clarke *et al.* 1977) (see Figures 1 and 2).

PAMPHLETS

There are four basic uses for the leaflet or pamphlet in the primary care field.

Firstly, in a similar way to the large posters, they can simply introduce a subject, relying upon the patient to seek further information. They should preferably be a single page, reproduced in large numbers, printed on one side only, and designed to state the subject and where further information can be obtained. Cost is usually minimal and they are intended to be thrown away once the information has been accepted.

Secondly, there are those pamphlets which contain information which may be referred to at intervals, and which can be kept as a record if necessary. Into this category fall those pamphlets containing immunization schedules, ages for developmental examination of children, dates for cytology checks and even appointment cards. The necessary information can also be accompanied by simple, even one sentence, guidance: 'Always wash your hands after using the toilet' or 'Please phone your doctor early if you need a home visit'.

Thirdly, the need to encourage self-care can be supported by issuing short printed, or even duplicated sheets with basic treatment schedules.

'In sickness and diarrhoea, medicine seldom alters the course of the illness, and may even prolong it. The accompanying schedule, lasting three days, will cure most attacks. If at the end of this time you are no

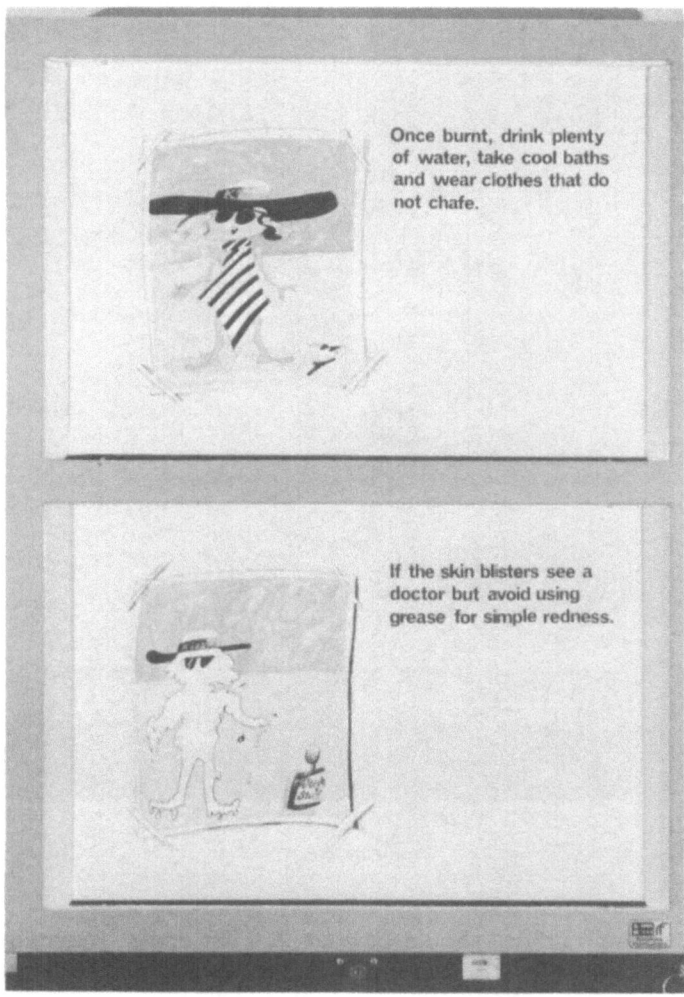

Figures 1 and 2. The Rotabine Machine. The poster at the bottom on Figure 1 moves after a delay of 7 to 10 seconds to the upper window revealing the next poster in sequence, as seen in Figure 1.

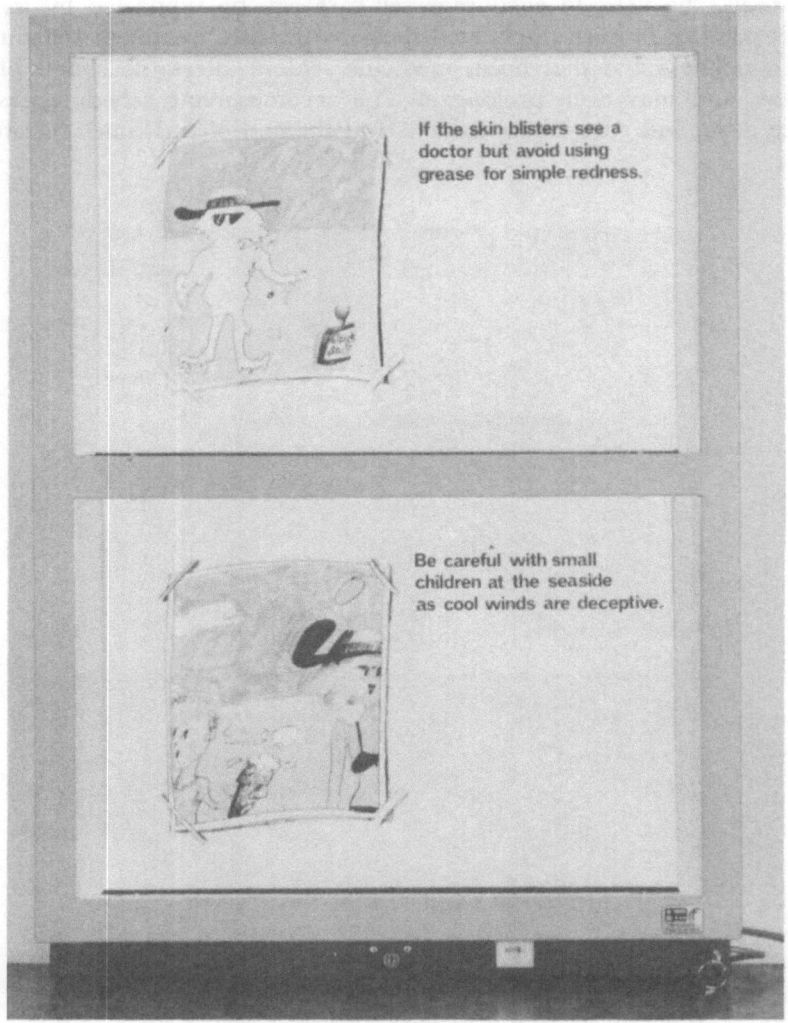

Figure 2.

better, a doctor's advice should be sought. First day . . . Second day . . .
Third day . . . '

Other illnesses helped by this approach are the minor upper respiratory
diseases, influenza, and joint and minor sports injuries. Such pamphlets
are for guidance and are intended for short-term retention. For this reason
they are better printed with a large sized type-face so that the patient with
poor vision can read them readily. A plain, tidy layout is adequate and
attractive in itself. If the sheets are duplicated, extra care will be needed to

keep them clean and tidy in appearance. Only one illness should be covered in each pamphlet.

Finally, there are pamphlets for retention as a source of reference and reinforcement after the consultation. Such pamphlets should reiterate in somewhat fuller form the points made, and aim to fill out the picture of the patient's illness. In this way, at second or subsequent consultations the patient may ask more relevant questions, and understand the management of the illness and what the doctor, nurse, or social worker is trying to do. These pamphlets will usually refer to long-term illnesses rather than minor or short-term problems. They should consider only a single disease and should probably be 10–12 pages in length. Suitable subjects are hypertension, bronchitis, ischaemic heart disease, pernicious anaemia and gout.

BOOKLETS

Booklets which accompany explanations given during the consultation can provide important reinforcement and may be offered to any reasonably concerned patient who is seen in practice. Short books, entirely in picture form, are said to have been useful in promoting screening campaigns in different areas; the strip cartoon has an appeal to certain people.

In the United Kingdom, the British Medical Association has published *Family Doctor* booklets on a wide range of subjects from alcoholism to the menopause, from the introduction of children to sexual relationships to coping with cerebral vascular disease. Patients frequently buy these books, and their availability in health centres and clinics rather than libraries is to be encouraged.

Production of these booklets and pamphlets may be difficult or costly, but a number of pharmaceutical companies and charitable institutes such as the Arthritis and Rheumatism Council now supply them free of charge. It is important that views conflicting with those in the pamphlet are not expressed by the doctor, without careful explanation to the patient. It is therefore essential to read any pamphlet from cover to cover before handing it out. Confusion is not the worst thing that can occur, distrust may also arise.

In the development of pamphlets of all sizes and types it is essential to gauge correctly the level of understanding of the patient. Here the language used is important. In areas with high immigrant populations it may be necessary to write, literally, in a different language, but in most contexts simple language should be used, avoiding jargon and medical terminology. It is equally wrong to fall into the reverse trap of writing in the vernacular. Such material is often not understood because of differing inflexions. It also loses authority by coming from a doctor whose use of such language is not expected. The appearance should be clean and tidy, colour may be helpful, it should be easily read, and the type-size must not be small. The suggested size for these pamphlets is octavo (20 cm × 10 cm) and must certainly be no larger than A4 (21 cm × 30 cm).

AUDIOTAPE

Since the development of the small, handy audiocassette, there has been much experimentation in its use for educational purposes. In the health education of patients however, the use seems to fall into fairly clear-cut categories. Before considering them, it is important to examine the requirements of the spoken word. The script for this purpose cannot be taken from a text book, but must be written as if in answer to spoken or unspoken questions. Punctuation and inflexions need to carry the necessary meaning in precisely the same way as the words themselves. It is of considerable value if the listener can identify the speaker, either a well known voice of authority – a television or radio newsreader for example – or, and this is obviously best, their own doctor or member of the primary care team. Preparation of the script will need not only a descriptive effort, but also some knowledge of the common questions arising in relation to the subject.

Perhaps the simplest use of the cassette is to answer set questions. In one experiment, patients in the waiting room were able to select a three-minute audiotape from any one of twenty-four questions. They could hear the answers to these questions over a telephone, whilst waiting to see the doctor (Clarke *et al.*, 1976) This exercise resulted in some 350 messages being played in a period of 7½ months. In spite of carefully planned changes of posters publicizing the telephones, this amounted to only a 2.5% use of the method by the 14 000 who came to the surgery.

Another trial used audiocassette tapes of some fifteen minutes in length played to groups of patients prior to discussion. The doctor, health visitor, nurse or social worker were then not placed in the position of the immediate authority and found the groups more relaxed at an earlier stage. Epileptics, diabetics, agoraphobics and patients with an ileostomy have found this helpful.

A further extension of the use of audiotape has been found to be acceptable to patients with chronic bronchitis, ischaemic heart disease or hypertension, who have borrowed a tape and played it at home. Here a twenty-minute recording is listened to by the whole family and has the advantage of involving the family in what is, after all, a family problem. It includes details of diet, weight loss or other required changes of habit. It has the benefit of interesting other members of the family in their own positions and the need for preventive action.

In some parts of the United States and Australia audiocassette tapes have been incorporated into the local telephone systems. In this way subscribers can dial a local bureau and receive a standard reply, on a pre-recorded audiocassette. Whilst undoubtedly it is helpful to provide factual information, such replies are unlikely to cover sufficient ground to answer the varying queries of subscribers.

Audiotapes in professional continuing and basic education are of established value. Where it is necessary to develop and deepen knowledge, or extend the range of group activity, as with voluntary groups helping in social welfare or first aid, more complicated audiotapes need to be prepared professionally, as do any accompanying slides. This is beyond the range of most primary care teams. However, the existence of these tapes should not be ignored as they are a sound and helpful basis for much health education work.

SLIDES

Photographic slides have a special value in practice. They are easily taken during the course of one's work, and quite apart from clinical disease, slides can be prepared about local facilities of all sorts. These are then used to illustrate talks, or to augment the consultation in a way that no amount of description can achieve. Every health team would benefit from a readily available camera. The impact of the written or spoken word is greatly increased when slides and photographs are shown to local groups or individuals. Slides used in instruction about self-palpation of the breast, or the use of the Wright peak flow meter by asthmatics, are but two examples of the value of professionally prepared slides.

If the photographer feels inclined to prepare slides for himself, particularly if they contain figures or numbers, he should be warned of the important rules concerning type-face and overcrowding of the slide. Advice on this is readily available from most medical artists, from Kodak pamphlets, or from specialist books on the subject.

The use of line diagrams, either as enlarged photographs or projected by overhead or slide projectors onto a screen, are of particular value to those who find the chalk and easel less easy to master. The explanation of cardiac infarction, hiatus hernia, vasectomy, or the introduction of an intra-uterine contraceptive device, can be simplified immeasurably.

MODELS

In recent years, cheaper, but still not cheap models of the spine, the female pelvis and other parts of the anatomy have come into vogue. That they add the third dimension is in no doubt. However, there is a risk of adding confusion rather than understanding to the untutored, who may find it difficult to orientate these models which may represent an unusual view of the body so far as they are concerned.

COMPUTERS

The computer, especially the new generation of microcomputers has yet to make its impact in family practice. At present it is seen as a sophisticated and efficient method for identifying groups of patients at risk for certain illnesses. It will record individual data arising in primary care so that detailed epidemiological information can be obtained not only on groups of illness, but on the natural history of individuals' disease. In this respect the careful selection of patients for invitation to talks and discussion groups will undoubtedly increase the educational benefit. The addition of a simple word processing programme to the microcomputer provides not only for the selection of patients at risk, but for the printing of a personalized letter together with an addressed envelope ready for posting.

It will thereby reduce the workload in circularizing those in need of such procedures as immunization, cervical smear or routine examinations and perhaps from simplicity allow further reminders to be sent out.

By rigid control of repeat prescriptions the computer will provide for many patients a much better basis for greater supervision by the doctor and perhaps they may learn improved management of their long-term illnesses.

If these applications, already in use in some practices, are in their infancy, the direct use of the computer by the patient is even less developed. However, there are programmes aimed at teaching patients the basic concepts of their illness and its management. These methods so far are extremely limited, not only by the need to possess a compatible computer but, of course, by the level of intelligence of the recipient. We must not underestimate, however, the computer applications in general practice and its linkage with the television set, which invades all our homes. It may well provide an almost perfect process for the provision of health education, if not at its best, at least at its most convenient.

VIDEOTAPE AND FILM

Videotape and film may be considered together. Both are of value when approaching larger audiences. However, videotape, unless accompanied by more than one monitor, loses impact, and of course visibility, if the audience is greater than ten or twelve persons, though a maximum of twenty can just about see a 28 inch screen if arranged in fan fashion. Film, on the other hand, is essentially made for the larger screen.

Perhaps the greatest problem of videotape is the high capital cost of equipment, though of course the running costs are lower than those of film because of the immediate erase and review facility. There are large libraries of film, whereas even after twenty-five years videotape libraries are only just beginning to appear. A number of doctors and nurses are interested in preparing and using their own cine films and videotape in their work. Audiences in general tend to compare such work unfavourably with the professional products with which they are familiar in their homes and cinemas.

Both fields are perhaps best left to larger organizations. The opportunity for borrowing and projecting their films and videotapes should not be forgotten. Many educational authorities and drug firms are willing to lend both the necessary material and the apparatus for projection.

It is seldom that any one method alone is of any lasting or worthwhile value. Health education is inadequate when practised in isolation and must be undertaken in a climate in which the patient is prepared to accept the nature of what is being said, and to act upon it.

The responsibility for providing this level of resource to awaken public awareness may rest nationally or locally upon those outside general practice. It is however, important that those in general practice should influence national and local bodies.

NEWSPAPERS

Daily and weekly national and local newspapers provide a forum for the public discussion of matters concerning health and the alteration of patients' behaviour. They also provide a means by which an individual's problems can be brought to the notice of the public, receiving discussion according to their newsworthiness.

The advertisement pages are a valuable method of promoting interest or concern about a particular health matter. The use of commercial advertisements may be one approach which has not yet been fully developed.

Articles on topical health matters, such as local outbreaks of food poisoning and infectious disease, may be used to give advice on prevention and first aid treatment or home nursing.

These may appear in regular columns or simply in the correspondence column. A letter from a locally known and respected doctor can help to generate the climate for behavioural change, or can support campaigns, for example, to keep dogs out of shops or to ban smoking in cinemas and concert halls.

The correspondence columns of newspapers provide the opportunity for a minority who feel strongly, to present their views and to have them answered.

RADIO AND TELEVISION

National radio and television programmes can provide, probably as no other medium can, a presentation of medical knowledge upon which public discussion and public awareness can be based. It is certainly true that the inclusion of medical matters is almost overwhelming in the television programmes of today, but the documentary production allows the public to become aware of developments and to enter into a discussion with some knowledge, however superficial.

In many parts of the world (UK, Australia, California) television programmes solely for doctors have been transmitted. These are tending to give way to older forms of communication as the necessary detail cannot always be included in the television programme alone. Too little use has yet been made of television for the purpose of public education and the involvement of people in their own health care.

LOCAL RADIO

The resurgence of local radio providing, as it does, rapid, up-to-date information on local, and therefore interesting, matters is a relatively unexploited field. Short documentary programmes are being transmitted. 'Is it cancer doctor?', a series of eight programmes is an example, (Radio Humberside, 1976). The need for accurate medical advice is almost insatiable. News and discussion programmes provide an opening for the family doctor of experience and common sense to educate a wide spectrum of people. There is much room for development.

TELEPHONE CALL-IN

Perhaps the telephone call-in, sometimes known as talk-back radio, has crossed the developed world faster than any similar programme. It is relatively cheap to transmit and enables a subject expert to discuss at first hand with the telephone caller, who retains anonymity, details of remarkable personal importance, which however, are often of value to a wide audience. The importance of these programmes has often been questioned, and there is some evidence that people who telephone call-in programmes have an uncertain pathology of their own. In my own experience (BBC Radio London, UK) the vast majority have genuine cause and ask questions which are answerable and of interest, not only to themselves, but to the wider audience. There is still a future for this type of programme, particularly if an attempt is made to link it with a documentary programme.

The extension of this approach to involve a panel of experts may go some way to giving a broader perspective, and in some ways a wiser one. It may be said, however, that if the person who calls obtains several answers which do not agree, greater confusion may result.

BOOKS AND MAGAZINES

Books and magazine articles, written and prepared from general practice, have a wide appeal, but their value depends upon the literacy of the audience, and the level and nature of the writing contained in them. Even sophisticated and highly literate people often find it easier to assimilate information in picture form. Such pictures seldom contain the detail experts demand. However the essentials can usually be conveyed more effectively by a clear diagram, than by the printed word.

In reviewing the field of health education in primary care, the role of the doctor must be seen to be first amongst equals. The final decisions on what is to be taught must be with the medically qualified. This is not to belittle the importance of the roles of health visitors, nurses, social workers or professional health educators. The need for education is not confined to the health care field, but must be carried forward in the schools, factories, offices and homes. No single doctor can bestride so wide a field, but the advice that is to be given to people in the name of health must be his concern. For this reason, if for no other, he must involve himself, and through him other health care professionals, at every stage.

In primary care the teams decide for themselves how best their work is divided. In the same way education will fall naturally into place. It would thus be expected that the health visitor would concern herself with children at home, in the school, and with their mothers and older members of the family. The nurse will best instruct at school, in the home where there is sickness, and at work. The social worker may be involved with relationships in the family, at work and where there is disability, and the midwife will be involved in the fields of pregnancy and family planning. The deployment of such a team may seem profligate, and so it is if coordination is not attempted. This is the role of the doctor, who is the only one to see the population not just in terms of morbidity, but as groups at risk.

References

1. Hugh-Jones, P., Tanser, A.R. and Whitby, C. (1964). Patients' view of admission to a London teaching hospital. *Br. Med. J.*, **2**, 660
2. Francis, V., Korsch, B.M. and Morris, M.J. (1969). Gaps in doctor–patient communication. *N. Engl. J. Med.*, **280**, 535
3. Pommerlav, O., Bass, F. and Crown, V. (1975). Role of behaviour modification in preventive medicine. *N. Engl. J. Med.*, **292**, 1277
4. Clarke, W.D., Devine, M., Jolly, B.C. and Meyrick, R. Ll. (1977). Health education with a display machine in the surgery. *Hlth. Educ. J.*, **36**, 100
5. Clarke, W.D., Engel, C.E., Jolly, B.C. and Meyrick, R.Ll. (1976). Health education in a doctor's waiting room. *Health Educ. J.*, **35**, 1
6. Meyrick, R. Ll. (1968). Medicine Today – an experiment in continuing medical education by open broadcast television. *Educational Technology in Continuing Medical Education.* pp. 63-6. (London: British Medical Association)
7. Radio Humberside (1976). The effects of a Radio Humberside programme, "Is it Cancer Doctor?" *Annual Review of BBC Audience Research Findings.* No. 4. (London: BBC)
8. Meyrick, R.Ll. (1969). Group viewing of "Medicine Today" television broadcasts – a small scale trial into subjective responses. *Television in Postgraduate and Continuing Education.* (London: British Medical Association)

Further reading

Jones, A.A.M. (1980). Health education to improve rubella immunisation in schools. *Br. Med. J.*, **281**, 6241, 649-50
Howe, H.L. (1980). Proficiency in performing breast self-examination. *Patient Counselling and Health Education*, **2**, 4, 151-3
Brody, D.S. (1980) Feedback from patients as a means of teaching nontechnical

aspects of medical care. *J. Med. Educ.* **55**, 1, 34-41

Essex-Lopresti, M. (1980). Illuminating an address: A guide for speakers at medical meetings. *Med. Educ.*, **14**, 8-11

Morrell, D.C., Avery, A.J. Watkins, C.J. (1980). Management of minor illness. *Br. Med. J.*, **1**, 6216, 768-71

Simmonds, D. (ed.) (1980). *Charts and Graphs*. (Lancaster: MTP Press, in association with the Institute of Medical and Biological Illustration)

Leathar, D.S. (1981). Defence-inducing advertising. *J. Inst. H. Educ.*, **19**, 2, 42-55

Oliver, M.F. (1981). The role of the physician in health education. *Hlth. Bull.*, **39**, 5, 296-8

Margon-Davies, A. (1983). How the Health Education Council can help. *Br. Med. J.*, **286**, 2358. 23

Ellis, L.B.M. (1982). Health education using a microcomputer. *Prev. Med.*, **11**, 212–24

Sloane, P.J.M. (1984). Survey of patient information booklets. *Br. Med. J.*, **288**, 6421, 915

Royal College of General Practitioners, Family Planning. An exercise in preventive medicine. Report on a Sub-Committee of the Royal College of General Practitioners' Working Party on Prevention. Report from General Practice 21. *J.R. Coll. Gen. Practit.*, August 1981. (Hutchinson, A: Secretary)

Royal College of General Practitioners. Health and Prevention in Primary Care. Report of a Working Party appointed by the Council of the Royal College of General Practitioners. Report from General Practice 18. *J.R. Coll. Gen. Practit.*, 1981. (February). (Chairman: J.M. Horder)

Royal College of General Practitioners. Prevention of psychiatric disorders in general practice. Report of a Sub-Committee of the Royal College of General Practitioners' Working Party on Prevention. Report from General Practice 20. *J.R. Coll. Gen. Practit.*, 1981 (February). (Chairman: Graham, P.)

Royal College of General Practitioners. Prevention of arterial disease in general practice. Report of a Sub-Committee of the Royal College of General Practitioners' Working Party on Prevention. Report from General Practice 19. *J.R. Coll. Gen. Practit.*, 1981. (February). (Chairman: Hart, J.T.)

Ruel, A. and Adams, G.R. A parenting group in general practice. *J.R. Coll. Gen. Practit.*, 1981, **31**, 496–9. (August). (7 young mothers met 21 times in 6 months for discussion of problems).

St. George, I.M. (1982). Is a tape-slide programme acceptable to patients in general practice? *N. Zeal. Fam. Physic.*, **9**, 77–8. (10 patients requesting vasectomy in survey: New Zealand)

Bryant, W.H. (1980). Patient education in the doctor's office: A trial of audiovisual cassettes. *Can. Fam. Physician*, **26**, 419–21. (Utilization of 12 tapes surveyed)

Cole, R. and Holland, S. (1980). Recall of health education display materials. *Health Educ. J.*, **39**, 74–9. (Survey of 2 weeks 1978: in health centre waiting room)

Stewart, M. (1982). Factors affecting patients' compliance with doctors' advice. *Can. Fam. Physician*, **28**, 1519–26. (Survey on preventive advice from 24 physicians: Nova Scotia and New Brunswick)

Andersen, N.A. (1982). Health promotion in general practice. *Aust. Fam. Physician*, **11**, 399–405

Johnstone, A. (1982). Validity in practice of the general health questionnaire. *Pulse*, **42**, 82. (1093 consecutive surgery attenders fill in GHQ)

Marsh, G.N. (1980). The practice brochure: a patient's guide to team care. *Br. Med. J.*, **281**, 730–2. (Brochure given to 262 new patients)

Morrell, D.C., Avery, A.J. and Watkins, C.J. (1980). Management of minor illness. *Br. Med. J.*, **280**, 769–71. (Dec. 1977–Dec. 1978: 999 individuals)

Pike, L.A. (1980). Teaching parents about child health using a practice booklet. *J. Coll. Gen. Practit.*, **30**, 517–9. (1978 survey)

Hill, D., Carson, N., Gardner, G., East, S., Gray, N., Heffernan, M. and Paget, N. (1979). Simple health education about breast cancer in general practice. *In. J. Health Educ.*, **22**, 25–9. (Six group practices in Australia)

Stewart, C. (1980). Patient education in family practice. *Florida Fam. Physic.*, **30**, 9–12. (Sample of 19 family practice residents surveyed for attitudes towards giving patient education)

Turner, J., Irwin, G. and Roy, D. (1981). Do patients read breast self-examination booklets? *Health Educ. J.*, **40**, 11–12. (Research in country practice: 303 women picked with random sample to read Health Education Council booklet)

Gray, M. and Fowler, G. (eds) (1983). *Preventive medicine in general practice*. Oxford General Practice Series 3. (Oxford: Oxford University Press)

Wechsler, H., Levine, S., Idelson, R.K., Rohman, M. and Taylor, J.O. (1983). The physician's role in health promotion: a survey of primary-care practitioners. *N. Engl. J. Med.*, **308**, 97–100. (433 physicians' responses analysed. 82 Gps., Massachusetts, June 1981)

8

Medical Records

EDWARD GAWTHORN (AUSTRALIA)

Medical records have been done, as it were to death, by various authors. It is hoped that this chapter will present a new slant on this apparently technical subject, which is, however, related to so many complex human needs. Have we mastered the technology, or have we become slaves to the systems of our own making? Such questions are well illustrated by a study of this subject from a humanitarian viewpoint.

To quote an example: the eighteen-year old, having been incorrectly labelled in her record as a paranoid schizophrenic, who bore the cross of this almost criminal error through long years of incorrect psychiatric management. This hopefully rare event (although a psychiatrist friend informs me that such is all too common) can be coupled with the everyday occurrence of the record interposing between the patient and the doctor to interfere with, rather than assist their interpersonal relationship.

During the past two decades we have mastered the technology. Now we must get back to being *real* doctors, using this technology only for the benefit of the people for whom we should care. It is in this spirit that this chapter is offered.

THE NEED FOR GOOD RECORDS

Why do we need medical records, what sort of records do we need, and how best should they be used?

The needs are amply testified by patients, staff, and doctors in practices which have changed to modern systems from old, narrative style history cards. Doctors will agree that such a change inevitably improves their clinical methods, by giving them the opportunity for a new look at their professional habits, and by aiding them in a logical approach to patient care. Patients are happy because they get better value from their visit, staff are happy with efficient filing systems, and consultants to whom the patient is referred, benefit from the receipt of good, well-documented case notes.

Broadly, the need for good records can be categorized into patient needs, staff needs, and general or community needs. Some of these may be common to more than one category, and some may clash, necessitating a balance between opposing goals. Important needs can be listed as follows.

Patient needs

1. That the information given is correctly recorded and retrievable when required.
2. That nothing is written in the record which may prejudice the patient's interests, and that only what is acceptable is recorded.
3. That privacy of the record is maintained, but that it can be communicated easily to other health professionals when necessary.
4. That health care programmes, such as immunization schedules, and other preventive care, be built into recording systems, and that a reminder system for follow-up visits, routine care, and immunizations be included.
5. That record systems assist patients to understand health maintenance programmes and their medical problems and to cooperate in the management of these.

Staff needs

1. To record each patient's attendance and the reason for that visit for medical, billing, and medico-legal purposes.
2. To facilitate data acquisition from new patients, and those presenting with new problems.
3. To highlight all important health milestones, including present problems and past history, and to structure these in a rapidly retrievable form.
4. To give priority in retrieval to the clinician's consciousness of such matters as the present problem list, current medications and possible drug and other interactions.
5. To provide information on allergies and immunizations.
6. To ensure a linkage between members of the same family group, and to other health agencies which the patient attends.
7. To assist communications in team situations (both intra- and extramural) and to facilitate the efficient use of secretarial and support staff.
8. To assist in research.

Community and other needs

Medical records must be tailored to the needs of the community being served and priorities must be preserved. It would be ludicrous, for example, for a sophisticated system to be developed for an unde-

veloped jungle region with scant health services and with a priority need
for improved nutrition and water supply. As such an area awakened to its
first steps in development, the first medical recording need would be a list
of recipients of immunization programmes.

Conversely, interesting examples can be given of the failures of Western
culture with its sophisticated development of both society and its health
services. Three of these are the failure of parents to bring their children to
free immunization programmes, the equally appalling failure of people to
attend for follow-up of major problems, and the failure of doctors to use
health recording systems effectively to their own advantage and that of the
patients whom they serve.

Other needs include flexibility to allow special requirements and
freedom of choice. We must never impose regimentation on people, but
proper communication between centres dictates the need for some measure of uniformity.

Medical records must be geared to necessary research programmes.
Whilst in a sense all records are used for research, special needs of units
may demand special records unsuited to general requirements. Because
family practice is often the only place where accurate morbidity assessment can be achieved, community research based on the local practice
should be encouraged, and therefore recording systems should generally
be designed to facilitate this.

The financial aspects of health records require consideration. What is
the prime and ongoing cost in terms of equipment, software and manpower? What benefits can be derived from such costs, and how can these
accurately be assessed in terms of actual improvement in health care?
Some benefits are obvious and easily evaluated, but others are not. The
cost factor must be related to the requirements of the system, and a
balance between cost and effectiveness is always important.

Ideally the community should expect that each individual have a health
record for life, following him wherever he moves, but with the increasing
mobility of modern society and the multiplicity of health services, this is
impossible to achieve without some national, or even international uniformity of standards. Here considerations of privacy versus expediency
emerge, and both the patient and his physician may justifiably fear the
intrusion of a government agency into the traditionally private consulting room. Again it should be stressed that the patient has an interest in
what is written and must at all times be given the opportunity to accept
this. There are many reasons why he may want to forget unfortunate past
problems. Equally important to his well-being, however, may be the
possession of such information by his trusted physician.

PRINCIPLES UNDERLYING, AND FEATURES OF, GOOD RECORDS

The first principle of any system is to satisfy the needs. All medical
recording systems should periodically be reviewed according to this

obvious concept and, if found deficient, should be revised or abandoned for an alternative which really does satisfy the needs.

The motivation for such a change deserves comment. It is true that once a system is established, it is difficult to change. It is also unfortunately correct that the software of systems is often designed by people incompetent to grasp the true needs of users, for example, printers, systems manufacturers, and government committees. Thus users have inefficient systems imposed upon them, with resultant failure to satisfy needs. It is also unfortunate that doctors sometimes cannot be motivated to update their records. Often a group of professionals will adopt policies acceptable to the lowest common denominator amongst them.

We must attempt to counter such problems by active participation in the design of systems, ensuring that outside agencies which serve us actually know what they are doing, and by an aggressive attitude to educational programmes directed towards the new generation of graduates. We must ensure that their demands for high quality tools do not go unfulfilled. Good records are as important as scalpels and drugs to good medicine.

Let us now illustrate the principles underlying good record keeping by dissecting the anatomy of a patient consultation and its follow-up.

At the time the appointment is made, or at registration, certain basic information is required from the patient for correct identification. This will be needed to establish the record for a newcomer or to retrieve from file the record of previous attenders. This basic information, which includes the name and record number, should be a feature of the outside of the record cover, and therefore easily available to the receptionist.

Records need to be kept in an efficient storage and retrieval system, in which they can never be lost. Having removed the record from file the receptionist will need:

*to initiate accounts procedures
*to identify family linkages and
*to identify special risk patients.

Features assisting these needs should therefore be placed on the record cover. An additional requirement for the record cover is identification of the year of attendance for culling purposes.

In building up the patient's history, a knowledge of other health agencies which the patient has attended in the past, or is presently attending, is required. Linkage to these, as well as family linkage, is important. In history taking, knowledge of the following is required and should be recorded:

*The reasons for attendance and therefore the current problems and their interactions.
*Important milestones in the past history.
*The psychosocial and family history.

*Information on immunizations and allergies.
*Anthropometric screening parameters, and notes on physical
   findings.

On review of this record, the physician should make an assessment of
the patient's problems and his plans for their management. This information should be clearly noted, and the patient involved in the process. Such
participation will enable understanding of the problems and facilitate
cooperation with the plans. A note on the patient's attitudes to this process
should be recorded.

A useful exercise for the reader is to consider and write down a list of the
absolute minimum data which should be recorded in family practice, on a
new casual or itinerant patient who could possibly eventually drift into an
ongoing association with the practice. It is interesting to note how often
actual records fail to reach this standard.

The author's own list is:

1.   Basic identification, requirements for billing, employment and
     qualification (or school grade for children).
2.   Reason(s) for consultation today.
3.   Allergies.
4.   Important past history.
5.   Present or recent medication or other health agencies attended.
6.   *Any other problems.*

Following appropriate examination the following is recorded:

7.   Positive physical findings.
8.   Any negative findings only if demanded by history or examina-
     tion*.
9.   List of plans mutually agreed with patient.
10. Arrangements for follow-up and by whom.

*The blood pressure is always recorded in adolescents and adults.

The list, expressed as an actual record, looks less daunting:

JONES Rosemary   22 Willow Grove   D.of B.   23/8/1958
Primary school teacher (1)
1968 Pneumonia (4)   Allergy penicillin (3)

20/3/82	"URTI" 3 days (2)	Fluids paracetamol (9)
	Nasal discharge (7)	Certificate 2 days
	Chest √Fauces √120/80(8)	
	Wants repeat OC (oral contraception) (6)	Microgynon 30 ED (9)
		6/12 (10)
	Dr. Bloggs. Smear 1981 (5)	
	Weight 52 kg (8)	

The information above the horizontal line will be transcribed to a Health Summary should the patient become a regular attender. The interrupted vertical lines divide the record into 'Findings' and 'Plans'.

In follow-up of a patient's problems, a recall and update mechanism is required. This enables retrieval, at any point of time, of accurate information on active problems and their current management. Recording systems should be designed so that items of importance are instantly identifiable at the moment of reviewing the record. We can then familiarize ourselves with this important data prior to concentrating on the patient unhampered by searching through volumes of paper or visual display units, both of which may distract.

Information requiring priority includes the following:
1. Basic information on the patient (name, address, category, and family structure).
2. When was the last consultation, and what was thought to be important at that time?
3. The active problem list, and current plans including details of medication and drug allergies.
4. What I am obliged to do this time (e.g. immunizations, health screening, necessary follow-up).
5. All other information which could be relevant to this consultation (e.g. past history, social and family history).

The important information for all future contact should be recorded on a suitable summary sheet, which is both updated and legible, preferably typed. *This is the key to good records.* Minutiae of past history, for example trivial events, or the fine details of major episodes, should not be allowed to clutter the record. The waste paper basket is an important adjunct to good record keeping. That is not to say that we should throw away our case notes; these may be needed for clinical or medico-legal purposes. But old case notes and piles of laboratory reports should never be allowed to interfere with important current needs.

In keeping of records and in filing systems the following principles should apply:

1. Records should be legible and easy to file and retrieve.
2. They should *never* be lost, and should always be updated.
3. All information on a patient should be kept in one place.
4. Family records should be linked in any system for family practice.
5. Special risk patients should be easily identifiable to all staff.
6. Active files should all be kept in the one place.
7. A culling system for inactive records should operate.

No system is perfect, but the features of good records can be illustrated by study of the Royal Australian College of General Practitioners' Health Record (RACGP, 1974). This was designed in 1974, and following clinical trials, in a five year period of marketing by the College since 1976, over

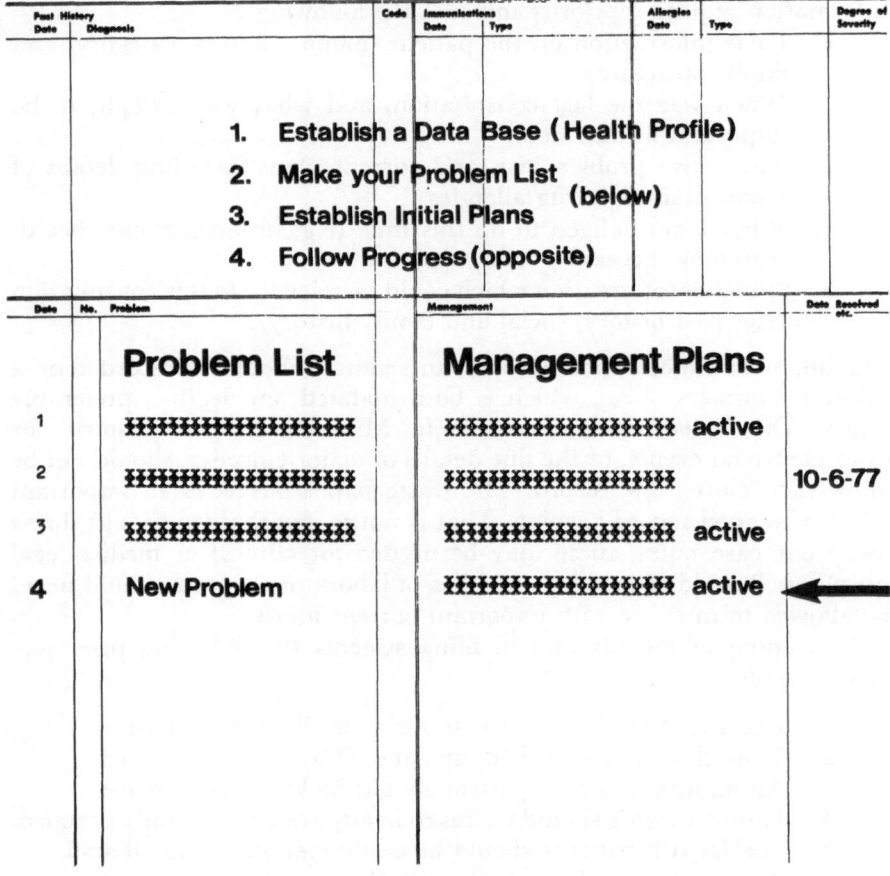

Figure 1   The RACGP Health Record

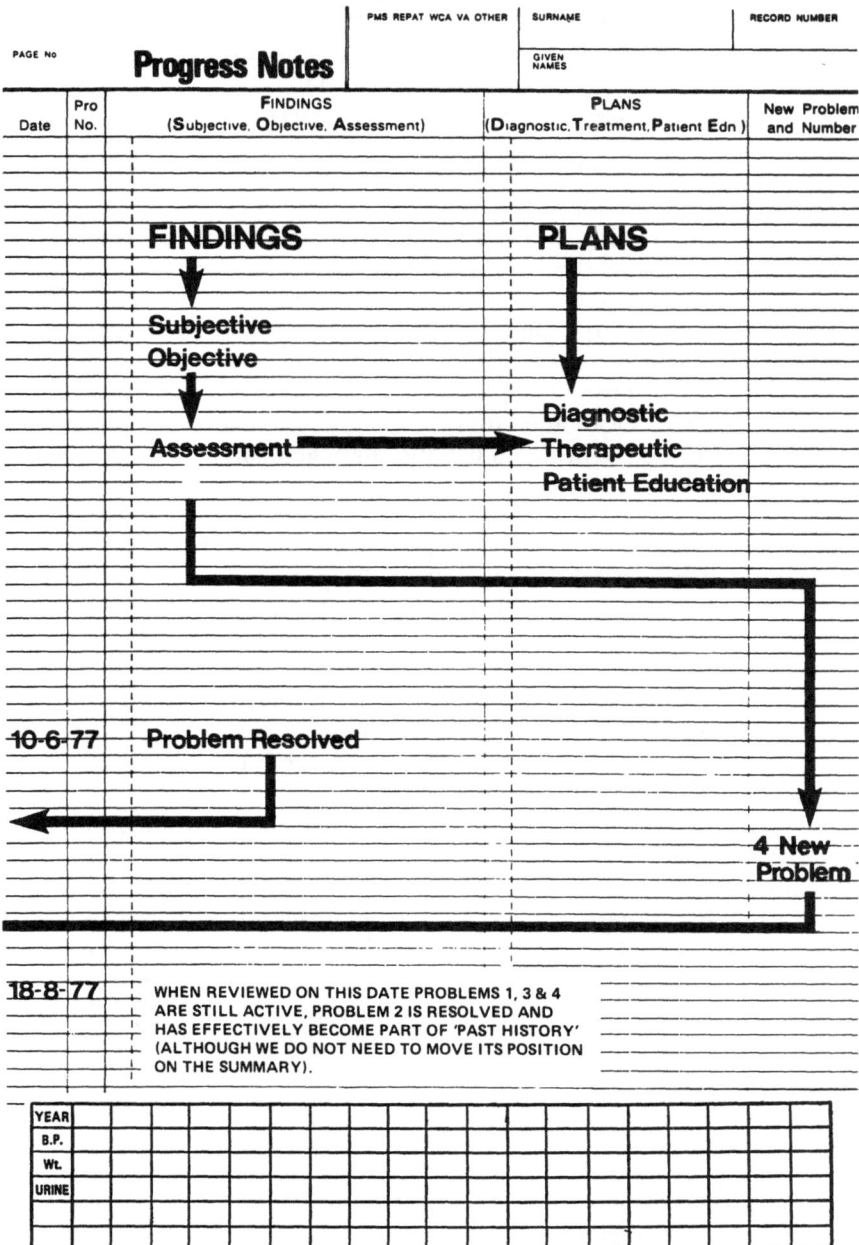

		PMS REPAT WCA VA OTHER	SURNAME		RECORD NUMBER

Progress Notes

PAGE No

GIVEN NAMES

Date	Pro No.	FINDINGS (Subjective, Objective, Assessment)	PLANS (Diagnostic, Treatment, Patient Edn)	New Problem and Number

FINDINGS

PLANS

Subjective
Objective

Assessment ─────────➤ Diagnostic
Therapeutic
Patient Education

10-6-77 Problem Resolved

4 New Problem

18-8-77 WHEN REVIEWED ON THIS DATE PROBLEMS 1, 3 & 4 ARE STILL ACTIVE, PROBLEM 2 IS RESOLVED AND HAS EFFECTIVELY BECOME PART OF 'PAST HISTORY' (ALTHOUGH WE DO NOT NEED TO MOVE ITS POSITION ON THE SUMMARY).

YEAR																
B.P.																
Wt.																
URINE																

50% of general practitioners in the country have purchased and installed the system. This wide acceptance leads the author to believe that it can justifiably be used as an example (see Figure 1).

The folder is A4 size, filed on its spine. Externally, space for name, family and personal record number, colour coding and year of attendance, 'at-risk' sticker, and family and hospital linkage, is provided. The opened folder features two small flaps. Printed on one is a matrix for annual weight, BP, urine testing and other data such as Pap. tests. There is no fixing of papers within the folder, so that currently used documents are kept to the fore. The left flap is designed to feature the patient's *Health Summary*. The right flap contains all other retained documents, with current *progress notes* or other currently used paper on top. Therefore the clinician obtains instant reference on the *Health Summary* to sections on basic identification, social and family history, past history, immunizations, allergies, and the active problem list and management; and on the *progress notes* to the details of recent consultations.

The Health Summary is the one non-negotiable component of the system. By its production the College has hoped to produce an easily photocopied standard which can follow the patient to his new medical adviser wherever he travels, and can aid the referral process to consultants or hospitals. In all other respects the system is flexible to allow for a wide variety of choices and needs.

The system is designed for doctors who orient their work towards health maintenance and where appropriate ascertaining patients' problems and their management. No system is problem-oriented; it is the doctors who use systems who should be so!

The progress notes are structured to assist these problem-oriented doctors. They give instant reference to details of current findings and plans and changes in these. Additional to these two documents, the basic patient kit also contains a *Reports Summary*, which forms an index to retained reports, as well as being a suitable replacement for large pieces of paper containing few words sent by such as pathologists or radiologists.

A full range of other software aids is also available for special needs. Some of these are listed hereunder since they highlight the additional components of any good record system.

Aids to data acquisition:
  Patient questionnaires
  Health screening forms
Paediatric Summary. This replaces the Health Summary in the care of children.
Obstetric care forms.
Flexible flow chart. This can replace progress notes in the maintenance management of chronic conditions.
Social profile. This can be housed with the Health Summary in

situations where a social worker is employed, or the doctor needs a detailed social history.

The RACGP has made every effort to make available proper educational programmes for doctors and staff in this recording system. We feel strongly that unless everyone in a clinic is motivated to the goal of good records, disasters can occur, and certainly the benefits will be reduced. A comprehensive handbook on the system is available to all potential users and the College employs assistants specially trained to demonstrate the system and assist in its installation. Two audiovisual aids are available, one tape/slide, the other a video cassette. The members of the Practice Management Committee of Council of the College are also active in assisting with problems. In summary, it is useless spending money on equipment and software without ensuring proper education for all concerned.

To return from the example to general principles, a word on patient's privacy is important. In medical records the principle of confidentiality should always be kept in mind, and patients' wishes respected. The potential for errors in this respect is multiplied proportionate with the numbers involved in keeping a record. There should always be a facility in any clinic for each professional to store information on a patient away from the general filing system. Important examples include the storage of the file of a staff member who is also a patient, and the storage of highly privileged information. It should also be the patient's right to insist that no record be kept, although it is important in such circumstances for the doctor to remind the patient of the possible dangers to future care, especially in emergencies, of such a course. Much depends on the type of information in question. No recording system should ever stultify the real needs of the patient through too much emphasis on confidentiality. A sensible approach to the question should be encouraged in patients and health professionals alike.

To summarize, the essential principles of good record keeping are ease of data input and retrieval, simplicity, completeness, flexibility, legibility, confidentiality, and reasonable cost-effectiveness in meeting the needs of the patient, the health team and the community.

PERSONAL HEALTH RECORDS

The accent of modern health care is that of self-care. The days of prescriptive medicine by professionals and patients obeying doctors orders are gone. Our patients now demand, and rightly expect, to be involved in their own care; our role being to advise, support, and to act as a resource for their own self-help and education process.

The logical extension of these matters in the field of records is the Personal Health Record. This component of the RACGP Health Record was designed in 1974. For obvious reasons this was highly acceptable to the majority of people, but doctors expressed grave misgivings, and it was not until recently that sufficient numbers have accepted the idea to inspire confidence in the future acceptance and viability of these records linked with the doctor's own folder.

Traditionally, soon after the birth of her baby, **Mother** became the possessor of a 'Baby Book'. During infancy it is useful in the hands of Mother, infant welfare clinic and family doctor. But, as the child begins to walk, it is cast aside.

Now **the child** may receive a Personal Health Record. In infancy it serves exactly the same functions, but it can be modified progressively for childhood, adolescence and in adults tailored to meet individual needs and linked with the doctor's record.

How many adults do not know:
  *when they had their blood pressure checked?
  *tetanus immunization?
  *smear test?
  *allergies?
  *what was important in the past medical history?
  *what medication has been prescribed and what they are **actually** taking?

With Personal Health Records they can have this information. In Australia and in other countries, the population is highly mobile. People often consult their general practitioner and also hospital outpatients for different things. Unless one proposed a national computer-linked system, the only way to keep track of health records is for the patient to carry his own whenever he attends any health agency.

In the RACGP system, Personal Health Records are contained in a plastic wallet designed to contain A5 size paper and folding to pocket or handbag size (155 × 110 mm). The wallet contains clear plastic compartments front and rear, and a clip suitable for all retained material. The forward compartment is designed to retain a short version of the patient's Health Summary, that at the rear for repeat prescriptions, health fund book, pension entitlement card or other similar material. The plastic clip contains any material suitable to the patient's needs.

Examples are:
  *Health Notes. The patient is encouraged to make **brief** records of important matters. Similarly the notes can be used by visiting nurses, infant welfare centre, or other professionals whom the patient sees.
  *Medication List.
  *Flow Chart. An important example of use is for a weight record.
  *Percentile growth charts.
  *Health education material.
  *Immunization record.

In the consulting room when both the doctor's and patient's folders are open, they can look alike. The patient can be encouraged to take part in the process of recording agreed plans, and repeat prescriptions are less likely to be mislaid. The whole process can be rendered satisfying to both the patient and his professional adviser.

Some possible problems must be mentioned. Examples are outlined below:

1. *The doctor feels that his status is eroded by patients having too much power, knowledge or control.* It is the author's belief and experience that this does not apply. In fact the reverse is the case where the doctor shows enough interest in his patients' welfare to introduce the system and encourage its proper use. It is true however that doctors may feel threatened if such a system is imposed upon them. Therefore an essential ingredient is for gradual introduction on a voluntary basis by doctors themselves commencing with groups of people with special need. Examples are children, the elderly, or people with chronic illness requiring long-term maintenance care.

2. *Litigation or other hazards arising from incorrect information.* There is world-wide debate on accessibility and ownership of doctors' records. Our own records can be subpoenaed to courts. The possession by the patient of accurate information on his health can make little difference, the advantages far outweighing this potential hazard.

3. *Confidentiality.* The patient has control over the record. It is for him to judge to whom it should be given. It is true that there may be potential problems when a patient wishes some past event to be unrecorded, especially for example, with a new marital partnership. In such cases the doctor can assist with the provision of a new Health Summary omitting the offending information with a suitable explanation to the patient, if required, on its potential future importance.

4. *Obsession with the record.* As a vehicle for communication, the records may lose usefulness if cluttered by a daily diary of minor ailments. However, there is an advantage if the recording of such a diary leads the patient to realize that they have, and learn to cope with, deep psychiatric problems. Generally it is helpful if patients are advised how to use the Health Notes with an accent on brevity and noting only things they consider to be important.

PROBLEM-ORIENTED MEDICAL RECORDS

The problem-oriented medical record (POMR) follows *problem-oriented doctors* in their logical approach to patient care. The record serves the real needs of doctors and patients. The essential components are:

   A DATA BASE from which we establish, where appropriate
   THE PROBLEM LIST from which is prepared
   MANAGEMENT PLANS which we follow by
   PROGRESS NOTES.

The *data base* begins with the first contact that a patient makes with a

health agency. Until its full establishment is completed, the most significant problem is the inadequacy of our data. Of course it is unnecessary to
write this down as Problem No.1, for we would begin with the error of
cluttering the record, but it is important to bear it in mind. This applies
frequently in situations where the patient uses our services for some trivial
complaint and clearly does not wish to establish a permanent relationship.
The mechanism of such situations may be analogous to a transaction at a
local corner store. On the second or third visit of such a patient we find
ourselves drifting into a permanent association, and realize the inadequacy
of our data base.

Such situations rarely apply in health systems where each patient is
required to register with a doctor, but certainly presents a problem where
complete freedom of choice by patients exists. It is important that we all
encourage community education, whatever the system, directed to the
importance of an ongoing relationship of patients with their family doctor.
Perhaps the best example which we can set is to ensure the adequacy of our
records, and our willingness to communicate them when circumstances
demand.

To return to the specific content of a proper data base, it should include
information on the following components:

*Detailed personal identification, address, sex, race, age, etc.
*Family, past, and social history.
*Present state of health including the patient's understanding and
 compliance with health maintenance programmes appropriate for
 sex/age group.
*Psychological data.
*Complete anthropometric and health screening parameters.
*Immunizations and allergies.
*Subjective and objective data on present complaints, including
 results of necessary special tests.

It is only practical that such a detailed analysis should be restricted to
patients committed to a doctor's care. In the concept of a health record for
life, the record starts before birth with genetic, social, and antenatal data,
and should be built up by a continual process of updating, coordinated
with accepted preventive programmes. Such a record would render
unnecessary the costly and laborious process of establishment of necessary
data for new patients, and of course some important information is often
irretrievable.

The **problem list** follows the establishment, recording and analysis of
patient data. It is the key to the whole concept of problem-oriented
records, and the moment of truth arrives as we challenge ourselves actually
to commit it to writing, having attempted to define all the patient's
problems. Unless we make this attempt, and succeed, we can never
honestly assume that we are properly caring for the people who trust us
enough, blithely to commit themselves to our care. How many patients, for

example, have we seen who are always coming to the clinic with symptoms? For many months we write copious notes and never really understand the problem, until the penny drops enough for us to realize a psychological reason for their host of trivial complaints.

What is a problem? Each doctor or group must decide, but again we must state that it is undesirable to clutter the list with trivia. The author's definition of a problem is:

*any condition which presents a diagnostic problem or
*an accurately defined diagnosis of a major condition or
*any recurrent minor condition.

Expressed in another way, we may say that a problem is anything which presents a diagnostic or management problem to us **now**, or could be useful information to any doctor seeing the patient at some distant **future** date.

Often we will need to record problems in descriptive rather than generic terms. This will specially apply to patients with psychosocial problems, and will certainly avoid such disastrous incorrect labelling as outlined at the beginning of this chapter. It is more important to record an accurate description of observed facts, than, relying on incomplete evidence or lacking specialist expertise, label our patients incorrectly.

The term '*problem*' is sometimes unfortunate, for it can vest people with a '*patient*' status, where none exists. For example, pregnancy is a normal physiological process, and health screening programmes for well people with a significant family history could hardly be classed as problems. Both will need mention on the problem list. It may be psychologically harmful to the patient to have it assumed that problems must exist, and perhaps the terms '*Significances*' or '*History Summary List*' might be more appropriate, although clumsy. However, the fact is that problems, like weeds in a garden, are here to stay and we must perforce accept them. Let us resolve to counter this unfortunate misnomer and always attempt to guide our people positively towards feelings of wellness rather than have them obsessed with disease.

A problem can be updated to change its status as time and further information permit. This is illustrated by the following simple example:

| DATE EVENT | WRITTEN RECORD | |
	Problem	*Management*
Day 1 First consultation. Abdominal pain. Primary diagnosis? Appendicitis. We decide to observe.	1. ABDOMINAL PAIN	OBSERVATION
Day 2 Patient febrile. Hospital-laparotomy, appendicectomy	1. ABDOMINAL PAIN APPENDICITIS	APPENDICECTOMY

In the above example, had we recorded 'appendicitis' on the problem list on Day 1, it would have been too much of an assumption. Had the patient recovered after this day, and subsequently moved to a new location, how would the new doctor know what occurred from this record. He could look for a scar in the right iliac fossa, or he could ask the patient! If you need to ask the patient, your records are useless, and the thinking patient may consider you to be incompetent.

We must emphasize that it is essential that a list of all the patient's active problems be reviewed by the doctor before the commencement of the consultation. Inactive or resolved problems are essentially part of past history. Of course we need to keep these in mind, but with a rating of lesser importance.

Finally, it is essential in defining a patient's problems, that the patient be involved. Where possible, we should only record things that the patient will accept, and certainly things that he will not accept must not go on the problem list. Such can be legitimately recorded in the assessment section of the progress notes, but the patient's problem list is a document designed to be the ongoing and communicable vehicle for his health programme. This statement highlights the need for proper two-way communication between patients and doctors. It implies that it is useless for us to prepare a product called a health programme tailored specifically to suit the patient's needs, unless it actually fits him, and he is prepared to purchase the product. Ultimately, if we fail to sell our opinions to the patient, as summarized in the problem list, we ought to offer to resign from participation in his future care.

Our **management plans** must be recorded specifically to fulfil the needs of the patient as summarized in the problem list. Many of the arguments which apply to the recording of problems also hold good for plans.

Before proceeding to management plans we should pause to ask ourselves several questions after we have established the problem list. Some of these are:

*How can the problems best be managed?
*Are any X-rays or other special tests required to establish a definitive diagnosis?
*Should the advice of a consultant be sought?
*What is the likely prognosis?
*How are the patient's problems likely to interact with each other or with those of other family members?
*What should the patient be told, and how best can I secure his cooperation and assist his understanding of the problems and the plans?

Often, if the problems are correctly stated, the patient himself will know what plans are required. It is much better for us to guide the patient towards an analysis of his own problems and their management, than to have our ideas on both imposed upon him. This especially applies to problems in the psychosocial field.

In purely clinical problems, with well-defined and accepted management routines, a reference to accepted recommendations for these is all that is necessary to record. An example of this is given in figure 2.

It is best to record only the major headings in management plans; with such details as drug doses which frequently change being left to the progress notes. Other minor changes in management can be recorded by an alteration in the progress notes, but as for the problem list, major changes in management should be recorded by restating the problem and its management.

The **progress notes** give us a work sheet for each patient's attendance. We can study each previously recorded active problem or each unrelated new one presenting under the following headings:

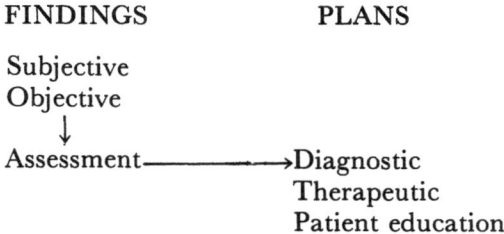

The diagram follows our logical processes of thought, and each active problem can be assessed, if required, in this way. It is important to the design and its uses that the headings be structured horizontally for each consultation date and vertically by category, for example, management plans. This gives us an easy method of comparison of clinical features and plans by a vertical visual scan, whilst maintaining a horizontal link between the groups on a time scale.

Any new problem discovered, or any change in status of a previously recorded problem, can be highlighted and added to the problem list, but trivial problems and their management can easily be recorded in the progress notes and need not be transferred.

Recording of details of medication deserves mention. It is important that these be highlighted and reviewed at each consultation to ensure that both doctor and patient know what is actually being taken and whether this is appropriate to current needs. This especially applies to older patients who become habituated and to people who fail to comply. It is the author's recommendation that current medication is recorded in **block capitals** at the top right corner of each page. This provides a fresh start, and an opportunity for review with the patient. Any later changes can be recorded similarly, a glance down the page enabling instant review of the updated list or dosage.

The Management of Gout

Diagnosis:

An acute monoarticular arthritis, usually associated with hyperuricaemia. Usually there are acute intense attacks of soft tissue or joint inflammation lasting days or weeks involving the first metatarsal-phalangeal and the midtarsal joints but not involving the spine or hips. Urinary tract calculi are common and often proceed the onset of arthritis especially in younger patients. A family history of gout is found frequently.

Blood screen and renal function tests point to the hyperuricaemia being due either to a blood disorder or renal failure. Diuretics, low-dose asprin and recent ingestion of alcohol all raise the serum uric acid levels.

Treatment of the Acute Attack:

Either: Phenylbutazone 100 mg tablets (rule of sevens) 7 tablets the first day diminishing by 1 daily to withdrawal.

or: Indomethacin 200 mg stat, 50 mg q.i.d. for 1 day, 25 mg q.i.d. the next day, 25 mg b.d. the day after that. Colchicine is effective when given as soon as the symptoms appear although vomiting and diarrhoea limit its use. It should be considered when other drugs are contra-indicated. Dosage: 1.0 mg stat, 0.5 mg hourly for 6 hours, followed by 0.5 mg 2 hourly until the pain is relieved or gastrointestinal symptoms appear.

Long Term Management:

Allopurinol 100 mg tablets. Single daily dose. Commence with 100 mg and increase until the serum uric acid level is normal. **N.B.** Lower dosage with patients with impaired renal function. To prevent attacks of gout induced by the allopurinol administer colchicine 0.5 mg t.d.s. Estimate serum uric acid monthly until allopurinol dose is stable then stop the colchicine and estimate every 6 months. Once established on effective treatment, diet and alcohol are not important.

Indications for Permanent Treatment with Allopurinol:

Problem 1. Recurrent acute gout (1 or more attacks per year). This includes secondary gout e.g. from diuretics.
2. Renal stones or tophi.
3. Possibly persistent asymptomatic hyperuricaemia (greater than 0.6 mmols – Litre)
4. Possibly a moderate hyperuricaemia as a therapuetic trial where symptoms are atypical for gouty arthritis.

– Dr. Julian Kirk,
Dr. Murray H. Bishop
Dr Bruce Morrison and Dr Peter Hatfield.

D4

Figure 2   The management of gout (Carson, 1980)

Some questions and misconceptions on POMR

Must I SOAP* every problem? Of course you must 'clean up' each active problem which requires your attention, but POMR is your servant – not your master – and should be used to help and not delay you. For example, if a patient has 6 or 7 active problems, most of which are well controlled or quiescent, it would surely be a waste of time and paper to fill a page going through the minutiae of recording SOAP for each problem. A good plan is to ensure that you revise the status of each problem when necessary, record essential clinical findings for comparison (for example, blood pressure in hypertension), and restate the status of each active problem at the top of each new page. Medication lists can then be checked and updated. It is often surprising, on this review, to learn the differences between the treatment that the patient has been ordered, and that which is actually being taken.

Why can't I write across the page? Of course you can! The vertical columns are for your guidance only, and to help you commence writing in the appropriate section. When a detailed history or case summary is required, naturally the whole page can be used. But then we should commence the next set of findings or plans in the appropriate column so that all can be compared by the simple act of looking down the page.

Aren't they really called 'Confusion-Orientated' records? No! Any system can become confused to the point of dissatisfaction if its users have not understood it. The better the system, the less the confusion. One only has to remember the muddled problems of old, narrative style histories to recall the difficulty of ascertaining one positive fact of importance from the laborious reading of many pages. It was often easier to start again by asking the patient to produce yet another bulky addition to the record!

Storage systems

There are three possible places where clinical information can be stored: we can rely on memory (our own or the patient's), we can commit it to paper, or we can use machines. A combination of these usually exists. For example, one word written on paper will result in instant recall from memory of masses of data. Our memories die with us, however, and are unavailable to the patient when we are on leave. Paper or mechanical systems must therefore be good enough to fulfil essential needs in our absence, and this is the essential test of any good system.

Paper storage

Some basic information on the principles underlying storage has already been given. We may now expand on this, but first it must be emphasized

*SOAP = *Subjective, Objective, Assessment and Plans*

that in the design of buildings and systems we must first consider the needs
of each consultation. These may be summarized in the following flow
diagram:

```
Appointment
made        A              B              C            D            E
  ↓
Patient  →  Record   →  Registration →  Doctor &    – – – →   Departure
enters      retrieved    procedure      clinical notes ↘        procedure
                                                  Secretary  ↗
```

In this situation, record handling has a possible five components (A – E
inclusive). The filing system should be kept near to the staff involved, and
therefore the building should be designed around the record. It is therefore
important to allow for possible future expansion or change.

It is essential, whenever possible, for the doctor to have each file open on
his desk **before** the patient enters. A useful project for the reader is to
assess the average time taken for each component of the filing and retrieval
process, and to assist in this process by meaningful *two-way* communication
with staff. This will often improve efficiency and allow staff more time to
fulfil their vital role of making the patients feel welcome, or for other
duties.

Active records should all be stored in one system, and each should
contain all the necessary information about the patient. For example, all
reports or consultants' letters must be kept with clinical notes. The storage
system for active records should also include files for itinerants or transient
patients. These will quickly pass to the inactive section if proper culling
procedures are used.

In storage systems it is important that families be linked. A family can
have one common folder, or individual members may have single folders
grouped together in the file. The advantage of family folders is attractive,
but this can be outweighed by bulkiness and therefore inefficient retrieval
within the folder. There is also the danger of accidental transfer of
information, such as pathology reports, from one family member to
another. Family folders also require alteration when there is a change in
family composition. In practices where the 'nuclear' family unit is
common, an outer jacket containing individual folders for each family
member is probably the best and safest plan.

Let us now study the detail of alternatives in the storage of paper
systems, which are listed hereunder:

1. *Size of the record.* There are many available sizes. The smaller the
record, the less storage space it will take. However, small records cannot
conveniently be structured – especially for POMR – and they are
inconvenient for storage of retained documents. A commonly used system
was 8 × 5 inch record cards. It was hard to maintain reports with these,
and seperate filing was necessary. There was also the problem of the
maintenance of an adequate health summary. The same size in envelopes

has something to commend it, for reports and letters can be stored therein, but these easily become bulky and frayed, and there is the nuisance and muddle involved in the unfolding and enveloping of contents. With these small sizes, good systems are not facilitated. The most popular modern size is international A4 in folders. This facilitates problem orientation, documents can be retained unfolded, and good filing systems are made easy.

2. *Methods of filing.* We must discuss alphabetic versus numeric, either serial or terminal digit filing. Alphabetic filing is useful for small practices with low record utilization. The advantage is elimination of alpha-numeric indices and the time taken for their operation. The disadvantages are the ease of misfiling, with its associated trauma, and the slowness of filing and retrieval, especially with commonly occurring names.

Numeric filing with colour coding of folders has many advantages. It is true that this involves the extra step of alpha-numeric referencing, but this is a small price to pay. It is reduced if patients are given a card showing their record number, and if appointment sheets are structured to allow space for these. Small alpha-numeric index cards or strips also serve instantly to link all family members for clinical or billing purposes.

Terminal digit numeric filing with colour coding of folders is recommended for all large practices or those with high record utilization rates. If ten colours are used in ten possible positions on the file, the total active file is divided into one hundred colour coded sections. If, for example, 9000 records were held, each section would contain only ninety folders, with each section equally balanced in number with all others. Should record No. 4682 be required, it is the forty-sixth record in bay eighty-two. The clerk may retrieve it in two or three seconds, almost the same time as it takes to press a computer key! Misfiling is impossible, for a misplaced record will shine like a beacon, and records can never be lost.

3. *Shelves versus closed cabinets.* Cabinets can be 'fire-proofed' and patients' privacy is more secure, provided that they are kept locked! They are slower to operate, however, and open shelves are recommended for ease of filing and retrieval. When staff are present, patients' privacy is equally preserved in either system. A filing cabinet is no less an obstacle to a burglar than a locked building.

There is merit in rotary filing shelves, which may particularly suit the design of some buildings. In all filing systems it is important to consider the maximum and minimum height to which staff will have to reach in servicing them.

4. *The bulky file.* This problem is lessened by good, ongoing summarizing procedures as the record builds up, and POMR is a potent prophylactic agent. Microfilm and microfiche techniques may be used to dispose of volumes of old paper which could only ever be required for medico-legal purposes, or on the remote chance that the detail of a very old consultant report may have a bearing on today's management. Should the facilities for microfilming not be available, one can always update the Health Summary by commencing Volume II of the record, and thankfully

consigning Volume I to the archives.

5.   *Culling and the transient patient.* We have already stated that culling should form part of any good system. To reduce stationery wastage, it is advantageous to keep the records of, say, twenty itinerants in one folder. These folders may have specially identifiable serial numbers, and such patients will feature individually in alpha-numeric indices (another advantage of numeric filing).

The files of transients should be kept in the same filing system as general patients, for they are easily retrievable, and some transients will be found

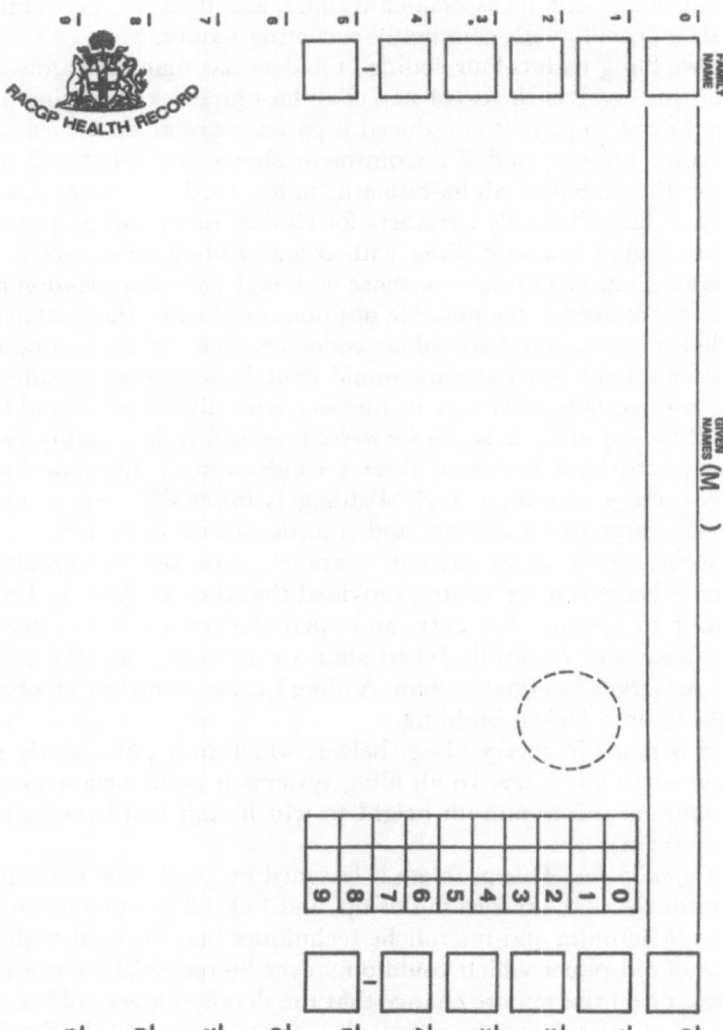

Figure 3   The front of the RACGP Health Record folder

to develop a permanent status with the practice. A culling procedure, preferably carried out annually, should be adopted, to remove from file the records of all those patients or families who have not attended recently. The assessment of the term 'recently' is a matter of individual judgement and will depend on factors such as the stability and density of the population, the availability of alternative health services, and the available

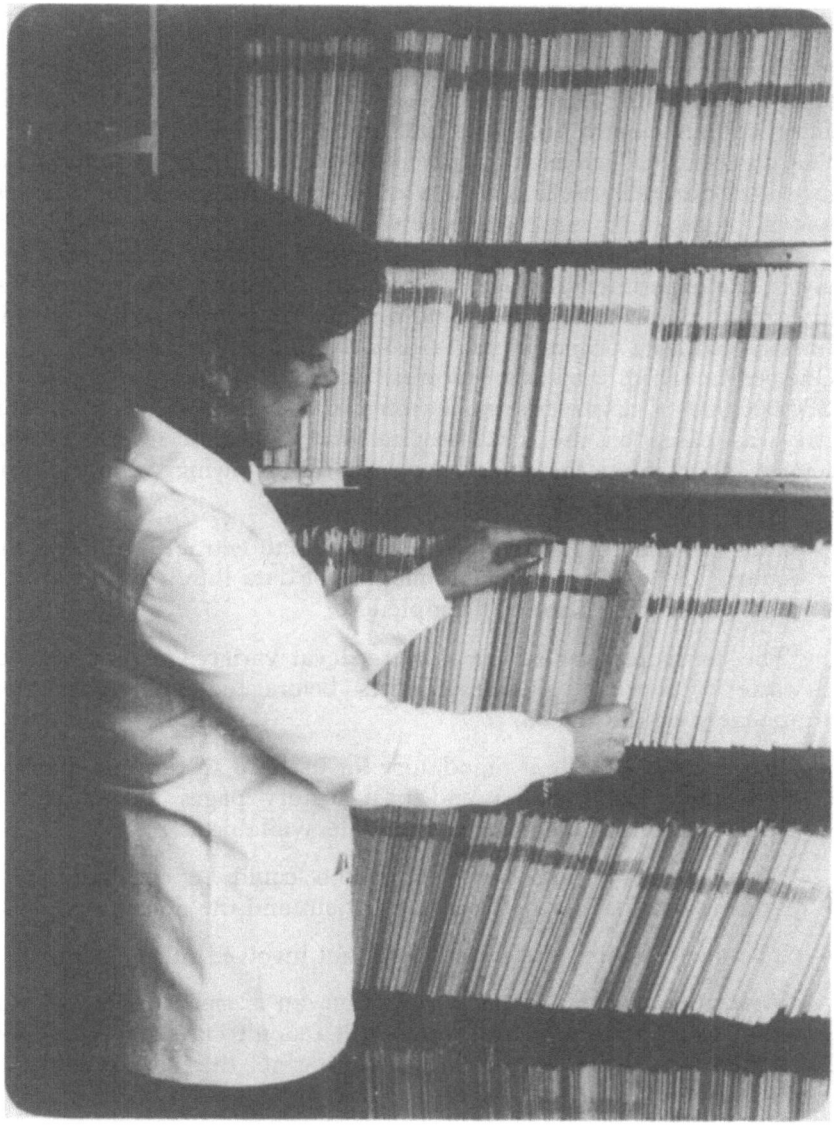

Figure 4 The RACGP filing system

space for an active filing system compared with an archival or inactive
location. Each clinic should therefore decide what is a 'recent' attendance.
Generally those patients who have not attended for three to five years
should be culled out. It is important to keep this problem under regular
review so that active filing systems are not cluttered with too many unused
records.

Computer storage

The subject of computers in medical records is more fully discussed in
another chapter, but for the purposes of comparison we can briefly
mention certain general principles now.

The computer offers exciting potential and challenge, but we must
ensure that our real needs are met as we enter this age of machines.
Previously computers were too expensive and too large to contemplate for
the average family practice, and programmes in some centres are still
really in the experimental stage. As computers become smaller and less
costly, this situation must change, and we must learn from past mistakes in
the design of future programmes. A classic example is quoted:

One centre, which the author recently visited, had spent the equivalent
of $30 000 000 of taxpayer's money on 116 000 patients' records. This
centre was based on the local hospital and linked to several general
practices. Apart from the staggering cost, the following problems were
apparent:

*Part time nursing sisters were employed to extract data from the
doctors' old cards, as the sole method of data input to the system.
This was admitted to be incomplete.

*The computer was of the slow retrieval variety, resulting in the
waste of several valuable minutes before required information
appeared on the screen.

*Programming made it mandatory for users to sit through displays
of detailed identification and past history pages before current
problem and management lists become available.

*Visual display units were large, and could be construed as a
psychological barrier between the patient and the doctor.

*The doctors using the system were not involved in its design.

*When the author arrived at reception, an exasperated doctor was
heard exclaiming to a staff member, 'I don't care how good it is
supposed to be, it is no good if I cannot get the information on a
patient who attended last Wednesday!'

Certainly we must learn from such mistakes.

On the other side of the coin, let us now list some of the possible advantages of computer storage over good paper records.

1. Associated billing and accounting systems are easily incorporated and are more efficient.
2. Staff time can be saved.
3. 'At-risk' patients can readily be identified.
4. Linkage between centres is facilitated.
5. Medical research programmes can readily be automated to obtain valuable information at virtually no extra cost, in terms of staff time and effort.
6. Information on drug interactions can be highlighted.
7. Associated educational aids can be incorporated, such as management programmes.
8. Comparison of results and graphic presentation of data is facilitated.
9. Automated prescriptions and referral letter writing are possible.
10. Information for practice management is readily available.
11. Reminder systems for non-attenders can easily be incorporated.
12. Disease registers are easy to keep.

Perhaps we should also list some of the dangers, not specifically outlined in the previous example.

1. Inoperative computers can be disastrous in medical practice.
2. Problems of confidentiality require study, especially with extramurally linked computers.
3. We must avoid the 'computer knows it all' syndrome.
4. Conversely we must avoid the 'blame the computer' syndrome as an excuse for our own mistakes.
5. There could be an increased danger of incorrect diagnostic labels being perpetuated. The relative difficulty of recording descriptive rather than generic names of problems makes this a reality.
6. With the pen we may heavily underline or use large block capitals for an important point. There is a 'sameness' with machine type.

Doctors who invest in computers should ensure that they fulful their needs and that they can be guaranteed continuing supply of software and ongoing maintenance contracts. If you want to buy a computer buy a good one. Two equally dangerous people are the computer salesman who makes false or misleading claims, and the recent purchaser of a machine who brags, possibly to justify to himself his large cash outlay.

With the advent of the 'mini' and 'microchip', the size and cost of computers is decreasing rapidly. At the present time, however, the idea of a combination of computer and paper records is recommended for consideration, because of the high cost of machines with the capacity to store *all* the medical records. Smaller machines can be programmed to record such items as appointments schedule, financial management, patients' basic identification and accounts, problem list, allergies, and current medication. A folder containing progress notes, consultants' correspondence, reports and hospital summaries, can complete the record. The progress notes may be used by the doctor's secretary to update the computer record when required. In the future it is important that all medical students become proficient typists!

The important point is that we must not allow our machines (or for that matter our paper records) to dominate our situation or destroy or modify that deep interpersonal relationship which should exist between our patients and ourselves. In summary therefore, computers have much to offer provided that we realize their limitations, and those of their operators. They must always, like any other tool, be seen to **assist** our needs in patient care.

CHANGING TO NEW RECORDS

The process of changing appears like an expensive and time-consuming ogre to those who may wish to do so, and so they tolerate the wasteful, inefficient muddle of old records. In reality it is easy, as our recent experience has shown.

Three phases of implementation of a new system can be described: organization, clinical, and health care. The organization phase includes all the steps taken after the decision is made, to the stage when all patients of the practice have new folders and stationery with the old notes and reports inserted therein. The clinical phase implies transfer of information from the old form to the new, and the health care phase means that patients involved with new records have commenced health maintenance programmes appropriate to their needs. The three phases will be concurrent to some extent, but are seperately described. Let us assume as an example a change from 8 × 5 inch cards to A4 folders filed on open shelves. The principles will be the same whatever the system employed.

Organization phase

As soon as the decision for change is reached, the following steps should be taken.

1. Ensure that the decision is clearly understood by all doctors and staff. It is important that everyone is motivated to the change and anxious to assist.

2. Choose a director. This could be a doctor or senior lay person to whom all staff (including doctors) should be responsible. The first task for the director is to ensure that all details are fully understood, and that alternatives allowable within the system employed are unanimously decided upon. People who go their own way in the use of any system can cause disasters.

3. Choose a changeover date. It is best to allow approximately three months before changeover, and, if possible, to choose a less busy period, preferably one when there are no staff on holidays.

4. Initiate an orientation and education programme. This may include precise typed instructions to all staff, handbooks, audiovisual aids, and visits to other nearby practices using similar systems. It is useful to remember that several alternatives exist for filing and usage. One can imagine the chaos created if one staff member **thinks** that he knows the filing method, but in reality uses a different method!

5. Order sufficient supplies (which should never thereafter be allowed to become exhausted), and make advance plans for housing the system. Should associated hardware, such as photocopiers, typewriters, shelving or an alpha-numeric index be required, order these early. Should internal building alterations be required, these should similarly be initiated.

6. If numeric filing is chosen, a useful plan is to commence a number register (serial numbers associated with names of patients randomly selected in order of presentation) for **regular** *attenders to the practice several weeks before the contemplated change.* Their cards, for example, could be distinctively marked by the doctor with a felt pen. Stationery is then prepared for those patients, in the new form, by staff during the 'prechange' period. On the weekend before the changeover day, all these old records can be quickly removed from file and slipped into the new folders, together with other associated reports. This means that the new filing system is established overnight for all patients who require high record utilization. In the author's own practice, 2000 records were so prepared, no additional staff were required for the change, and on the first day the staff were presented with an established system upon which they could build.

7. Just prior to changeover it is again important that all staff know how to prepare and colour code folders and insert new stationery.

8. On and after the changeover date it is necessary to allocate a new folder to each new patient attending, and at the same time to ensure continuing build-up of the numbers register and the alpha-numeric index. A decision is required on families. In the case of a practice with a stable population, it is efficient to prepare new folders for all members of the family when the first family member attends. However, this may be wasteful of much stationery in districts with mobile populations, or where there are several alternative practices. In each case where a new folder is prepared, the old records and associated reports for the patient should be retrieved and placed in the new file. The organization phase is deemed complete when nearly all patients of the practice have a folder, new basic stationery, and old records inserted. In practice, this has been found to take approximately six months from the changeover day, and reports from Australian practices have indicated that the employment of extra staff has usually been unnecessary.

Clinical phase

The *clinical phase* is largely up to the doctors. It is important to ensure that this proceeds smoothly without too great an erosion of the valuable time of those concerned. It is too easy for doctors to fall into the trap of trying to

CLINIC NAME

Health Profile '76 – PART I

PATIENT'S QUESTIONNAIRE

RECORD NUMBER

DATE

INSTRUCTIONS: *A complete medical history is important for you to obtain good health care. Please complete details on both sides of this form. If there is anything you do not understand please record a query (?). All information given is strictly confidential. Please feel free to tell the doctor anything you cannot write down. Please print in BLOCK CAPITALS, one letter or number per square.*

1. IDENTIFICATION

Mr/Mrs/Miss	Surname:
Given Names	Given Names:
Address	Telephone: Home:
	Business:
	Postcode:
Date of Birth — Day Month Year — Country of Birth	
Marital Status — Sex — Next of Kin	
Occupation — Religion	
Employer or School	Blood Group — Rh

2. SOCIAL PROFILE Please indicate (✓) where appropriate, or briefly state answers.

Do you take (✓)	What Form and Quantity	Are you an (✓)	Do you live in a (✓)	How many	No.	Please State Relationship to Head of Family (212)
200 Alcohol	201	202 Ex-Drinker	206 House 208 Flat	210 Rooms		
203 Tobacco	204	205 Ex-Smoker	207 Unit 209 Other	211 People		
213 Please State Past Occupations			214 Please State Hobbies Sporting or Social Activities			

3. FAMILY HISTORY This is important to your medical history. Please indicate (✓) if any of your family suffered or died from the following:

		Paternal Grandparents Male (1)	Female (2)	Maternal Grandparents Male (3)	Female (4)	Father (5)	Mother (6)	Brother (s) (7)	Sister(s) (8)	Son(s) (9)	Daughter (s) (10)	Other(1) (11)	Other(2) (12)
Heart Attack	(301)												
Blood Pressure	(302)												
Cancer	(303)												
Stroke	(304)												
Cerebral Tumour	(305)												
Mental Disease	(306)												
Suicide	(307)												
Diabetes	(308)												
Pneumonia	(309)												
Tuberculosis	(310)												
Asthma	(311)												
Anaemia	(312)												
Leukaemia	(313)												
Haemorrhage	(314)												
Kidney Disease	(315)												
Accident	(316)												
Old Age	(317)												
Age (approx.) at Death	(318)												

4. SYMPTOMS. PATIENTS Please list any present problems. | DOCTORS USE ONLY

RACGP © 04/2A

Figure 5   RACGP Health Data Base

5. PAST MEDICAL HISTORY Please indicate (✓) or fill in last 2 digits of year where appropriate if remembered.

Were you born with any Serious Abnormalities of	(✓)	Have you ever had Serious Disorders or Diseases OR YOUR	(Year or✓)	OR SUCH AS	(Year or✓)	OR RELATING TO	(Year or✓)	Have you ever Suffered from	(Year or✓)
501 Heart		509 Eyes		525 Convulsions		541 Breasts		557 Chest Pain	
502 Lips		510 Ears		526 Migraine		542 Uterus		558 Chest Tightness	
503 Palate		511 Nose		527 Glaucoma		543 Tubes		559 Breathlessness	
504 Eyes		512 Throat		528 Melanoma		544 Ovaries		560 Palpitations	
505 Ears		513 Teeth		529 Diabetes		545 Vagina		561 Swollen Ankles	
506 Hips		514 Bones		530 Gout		546 Cervix		Or Been Told That You Had —	
507 Spine		515 Joints		531 Pneumonia		547 Penis		562 Heart Murmur	
508 Others		516 Skin		532 Asthma		548 Testicles		563 Angina	
		517 Muscles		533 Ulcer:stomach		549 Prostate		564 Coronary Disease	
		518 Nerves		534 Duodenal		550 Bladder		565 Myocardial Infarction	
		519 Liver		535 Hepatitis		551 Kidney		566 Serious Blood Clots	
		520 Spleen		536 Tuberculosis		552 Adrenal		567 High Blood Pressure	
		521 Pancreas		537 Typhoid		553 Pituitary		568 Rheumatic Fever	
		522 Gall Bladder		538 Hydatid		554 Venereal disease		569 Endocarditis	
		523 Bowel		539 Osteomyelitis		555 Circulation		570 Nephritis	
		524 Thyroid		540 Hernia		556 Arthiritis		571 Scarlet Fever	
								572 Mental Disease	

Year	Have you ever had any other Serious Conditions, Illness, Operations or Accident?	X Rays and other Tests	
573		Year	Type and Result
574			581
575			582
576			583
577			584
578			585
579			586
580			587

Year	FEMALES ONLY — Please list in order all pregnancies or miscarriages giving details of any complications e.g. Toxaemia, Transfusion, Instruments etc.	Contraception
588		596 Past
589		
590		
591		
592		597 Present
593		
594		
595		598 Date of Last Smear Test

6. IMMUNISATIONS & ALLERGIES

Immunisations			Allergies — Any Severe Reactions		
Type	Last Yr.Rec.	Please List Other Types	Types	(✓)	Please List Known Allergies Here —
601 Tetanus			620 Drugs		
602 Smallpox			621 Antibiotics		
603 Cholera			622 Bites		
604 Rubella			623 Stings		
605 Typhoid			624 Food		
606 Other			625 Other		

7. MEDICATION OR DRUGS Please Print Name of any Drug or Medication you have been or are taking regularly.

	Example	A	S	P	I	R	I	N		(✓)	I have been taking this medications for (years) 0-1, 1-5, 5-10, 10
701											
702											
703											
704											
705											
706											
707											
708	Are you, or have you ever been addicted to Drugs						Yes	No	If 'Yes' Name Drug(s)		

8. OTHER HEALTH CARE Are you Attending Any Hospital or Other Clinic. If so Please State:

Name of Institution	Reason for Attendance	Record Number-If known

convert everyone seen in the first week and to become so far behind with their work as to be disillusioned, and to not convert anyone thereafter.

It is recommended that each doctor sets himself a target of say, twenty completed conversions each week. He will have finished the process with all his patients in approximately two years. It is further recommended that doctors select first for conversion those people who require full clinical assessment at the time. Examples are new patients, old patients with major new problems, or regular patients on maintenance programmes for important disorders (for example, hypertension, diabetes and so on). When a patient requires referral to a consultant, his record should be converted, for the letter of referral can be' improved by attaching a photocopy of a good, typed Health Summary. Later the doctor will find time to convert all patients on sight. There is much satisfaction to be derived from watching the build-up of well-prepared records.

In the phase of clinical conversion it is recommended that the patient's interest be engaged in the new record. Often a review of the old notes in the patient's presence will result in his volunteering important details of past history or family problems which hitherto have been unsuspected. A rewarding addition to the data base may result if each patient for clinical conversion is handed a suitable questionnaire for completion at leisure at home in collaboration with his family (see Figure 5). Important contributions to the patient's record at this time may also be derived from contact with other health care agencies which are attended. Generally it is essential that this task should be properly completed once it is attempted. With increasing utilization of good records, and with the ease of communicating health summaries, once performed for each patient, the task should never need repetition, wherever the patient may go.

Health care phase

The *health care phase* is probably the ultimate objective in the change to good records. The day of episodic patient patching should be gone with the realization that programmes of health maintenance are far more important than preoccupation with disease. Having converted the record clinically, we are finally in a position to assess the patient's problems or potential for these, and to undertake whatever programmes are appropriate.

Because the health care phase is ongoing, it is facilitated by the provision of good records, without which it is difficult to achieve.

Some general problems regarding conversion deserve mention. These are largely concerned with the education of doctors to use properly the systems which they install, and especially to orient themselves towards patients' problems. It is no use establishing a new filing system if you never complete the associated Health Summary. However, we must concede that it is sometimes difficult to change lifetime habits, especially in older doctors. What is important is that we must ensure that the new generation of doctors are trained to the real needs of patients and recording of their problems, and that they are given the recording tools appropriate to these needs.

THE USE OF RECORDS TO AUDIT PROFESSIONAL STANDARDS

Part of this concept is new and considered by some to be threatening. Part is as old as medicine and its record keeping, and acceptable to all. Let us consider the five sorts of people who could be involved with the audit of records.

Oneself. For as long as records have been kept, doctors have been able to audit themselves, when, with the advantage of hindsight, they have reviewed what was previously written.

The patient. Again this is a continuous and long-accepted process in situations where free, two-way communication exists between the patient and the doctor, the medical record being compiled in the presence of, and discussed with, the patient.

The 'friendly' partner or associate. Our partners, assistants, locums and trainees, all of whom use and review our records, when they subsequently discuss the interesting cases which have been shared, all play a part in audit. This is an acceptable and time-tried process.

The 'friendly' consultant to whom the patient is referred. The referral letter is part of the medical record, for it is an extract therefrom, and so is the reply. A process of audit by this method cannot be open to question.

'Big Brother', 1984, and all that! Here we have the contentious question.

In most countries in the world there is justifiable concern about the continuing education of doctors, and, depending on the medico-political system which exists, more or less accent on concomitant periodic assessment. To let a doctor loose on society by registering him in 1950 and to do nothing to ensure his continuing competence in 1980 is unthinkable to the community and its health planners. There is no doubt that the medical record **can** be used as a tool in the hands of the assessor, and of course the better the record, the easier it is to assess. Conversely, we should state that the worse the record, the more likely there will be failure to reach acceptable standards. The threat of assessment by review of records should never be used as an argument for the maintenance of antiquated methods.

The whole subject of peer review has been the core of much debate in medico-political circles. The author has no wish to enter this debate. It can be stated simply without fear of contradiction that the better the record, the greater the likelihood of the competence of its writer, and of there being a real bond of trust between the doctor and the most important person of all, **the patient**.

References

1. Royal Australian College of General Practitioners (1974). *Health Record System.* (Melbourne: RACGP)
2. Carson, S. (1975). *A Manual for General Practice.* NZ Edition. (Auckland: Beecham Research Laboratories)
3. Carson, S. (1980). *A Manual for General Practice.* Australian Edition. (Melbourne: Beecham Research Laboratories)

9
Group Practice Management

B. LESLIE HUFFMAN JR. (USA)

PRINCIPLES OF GROUP PRACTICE

The early pioneers in medicine, independent in spirit and few in number, were loners. Solo practice was the general rule.

The team approach to the practice of medicine is a product of modern times. No longer is it conceivable that one physician can be the embodiment of total health care. Today, medicine is a shared responsibility, involving physicians of all specialities as well as those in the allied health professions. The present group practice concept is an outgrowth of that realization.

There are other reasons for the increasing popularity of group practice other than the enormity of the task and the need for shared responsibility. Principal among these is quality of life. Even physicians of early times realized that full time responsibility for their practice was onerous. When other physicians were available, they would cover for each other in order to have some time for themselves and their families. Such coverage arrangements today are quite formalized and generally well accepted by patients. Although this can be accomplished through an agreement among a number of solo practitioners, it is most effective in the group practice situation where group liability is most keenly appreciated.

Professional enrichment is another asset of group practice. The day-to-day stimulation of the exchange of ideas with peers in your own specialty and with colleagues in other specialties contributes to your own knowledge and expertise. Some groups formalize continuing medical education more than others by holding regular meetings to discuss interesting patient problems together. Many require that a specific portion of each year be spent in continuing medical education efforts. In most of the groups in our part of the world, each doctor has four weeks vacation and two weeks for postgraduate education every year.

With these advantages, it is not surprising that a majority of our family practice residency graduates now enter some form of group practice. Many of them are moving into underserved areas where solo practitioners formerly were unable to cope with the medical needs of the population and still have any time for themselves. Geographic distribution definitely has been affected by the trend toward group practice.

Whether our graduates form their own group or join an established group, there are certain principles which help assure their success:

1. Whatever the *agreement,* **be sure it is in writing**. The details of a handshake are too easily forgotten. Include specifics in regard to compensation, time off, fringe benefits, overhead expenses, buy-in, dissolution, retirement and death.

2. *Compensation* should be based principally on productivity with a substantial guaranteed minimum at the start. Keep fixed distribution of profits to a minimum. A good workable ratio is twenty percent equally divided among all associates and eighty percent according to productivity.

3. *Vacation and fringe benefits* such as health insurance and pension, and profit-sharing should be made available to all associates on an equal basis.

4. *Time off for continuing medical education* should be stipulated. Two weeks per year is customary.

5. *Overhead expenses* should be based on productivity generally, if all associates are working full time. If one associate wishes to restrict his practice for some reason, there may need to be some adjustment for fixed overhead expenses.

6. Regardless of the group structure – whether partnership or corporation – a *value* should be agreed upon in regard to equipment, facilities and accounts receivable. After a provisional period of time, usually one year, a new associate should have an opportunity to buy into the group on an equal basis. Payment should be deducted from his compensation over an extended period of time.

7. Finally, provision for the *dissolution* of the group, or the death or retirement of one of its members should be included in the original agreement. This necessitates concurrence on the value of a share and the method whereby it will be paid. This valuation should be updated annually.

8. The actual *legal framework* of a group must depend on the current law of the land. The advice of both an attorney and a certified public accountant should be sought. Most large groups in the United States are incorporated, because of tax advantages.

GROUP SIZE AND CONSTITUENCY

Although there are other considerations, the geographical location of a group is the single most significant determinant of its size and constituency. In a remote rural area, a group composed only of family physicians could support one physician for each two thousand five hundred people. In the same area, a mixed group ideally would contain one member from each major specialty – at a minimum, an internist, a paediatrician, an obstetrician, and a surgeon. To support four such physicians, the area would have to have at least fifteen thousand patients. Moreover, unless each of these specialists is willing to cover another specialty area, none of the doctors would have coverage for time off. Generally, if a mixed group has a patient population large enough to support two in each specialty, it has some assurance of success.

The variety of specialty mix possible is limitless. However, my personal prejudice is in favour of single specialty groups, not only because of internal group coverage, but also because of the dissatisfactions that arise in mixed groups over the productivity differences in the specialties. For example, a single procedure for a surgeon might take several days in the office for a family physician or paediatrician or internist to equal financially.

There is a saying in American folklore that two can live as cheaply as one when considering the advantages of marriage. However, this does not apply to medical 'marriages' at all. Although some economies are realized by staggering hours to share the same space, and purchasing in large quantities, in general the larger the group, the greater the costs involved. Groups of four or more require a full time office manager and a head nurse. For this reason, groups of three doctors may be slightly less expensive. For the same reason, groups of five may be more economical.

OFFICE MANAGEMENT

Currently I practice in a four family physician corporate group. We plan to expand to five in the near future because this will enable us to better utilize our present staff and office space to economic advantage, and to provide better depth of coverage for time away from the practice for each of us. We practise in a suburban location and serve approximately eighteen thousand patients with the help of our ancillary health professionals.

Management of such a group requires the services of an office manager full time, and a head nurse. In addition, we employ a medical consulting firm with whose advice and counsel our practice group was incorporated. As a general rule, our regular management consultant visits the office every other month for two days to review current problems with our office manager, to interview our personnel to ascertain any difficulties there, and to meet with each doctor separately. Also, we hold a corporate meeting while he is present. Both the office manager and head nurse attend this dinner meeting and contribute significantly to its success.

Throughout the year, our medical management firm prepares monthly operating statements and net worth statements for the corporation and for each individual doctor. In order to provide these, all transactions are monitored and entered on their computer. With this information, all necessary corporate and personal tax forms are completed. Collections are monitored and our office manager assisted in follow-up. Overhead expenses are watched closely and compared to similar offices as to performance. Fees are adjusted accordingly. Advice about investments and pension and profit-sharing is offered.

If such a medical management firm were not available, we would employ a certified public accountant and programme our own computer to perform the same financial data functions.

Our office manager is responsible for all the business aspects of the practice. She conducts all job interviews. Job descriptions are prepared and updated with the advice of our management consultant. The office manager determines the business office work schedule, monitors time cards for all personnel, and submits payroll data to the management consultant for the bi-weekly payroll. All expenses are reviewed regularly and cheques prepared for our signature. Accounts receivable are aged, reviewed with the doctor concerned, and collection procedures followed up. Not only is she responsible for the work of the receptionist, telephone operator, two computer operators, and the file librarian, but she also must be able to function in any of these areas herself in an emergency. She consults with the head nurse on matters concerning the nurses and medical assistants, and reviews our budget with her for the purchase of supplies.

All personnel problems are discussed at length with the physician who is acting as business manager for the corporation. The office manager not only is responsible for all hiring, but ultimately is charged with the responsibility for all firing as well.

Finally, she keeps track of business office supplies and equipment maintenance, and makes all necessary purchases.

The head nurse is in charge of four full time nurses, four full time medical assistants, a part time nurse and a part time medical assistant. She conducts their job interviews and reviews their job descriptions with them. She assigns their duty schedule and reviews their time cards with the office manager.

Since our head nurse also serves as my own nurse clinician, she has divided many of her duties among the other nursing personnel. While she herself orders drugs and new diagnostic and therapeutic equipment, other nurses monitor different supply areas and prepare patient summaries for insurance companies.

The head nurse keeps all the appointments with supply house representatives herself, and meets with pharmaceutical representatives on a regular schedule.

Ultimately, the efficient office management of nursing personnel depends on the availability of an experienced and competent head nurse.

In any practice group, one of the physicians should be appointed to oversee the office manager and the head nurse. They need to have a specific individual available for consultation, assistance in job interviews, settling intramural disputes and signing bank drafts. This is a responsibility which we rotate in our group on an annual basis. Even though one may be superior to another in dealing with such business matters, it is an experience all should share.

SYSTEMS IN GROUP PRACTICE

Patient flow

There are a number of systems which contribute to the efficiency of any medical group practice. However, in the selection of any of these, we must not lose sight of the fact that the patient is our primary concern.

As my own group expanded from one to four physicians, our first approach was to add more people to receive patients, answer the phone, take messages, handle payments, post laboratory work, and file. The group appointment book grew larger and more unmanageable and had to be custom printed at great expense. Communication between the enlarged office staff and expanded nursing staff often failed, resulting in appointment errors and dissatisfied patients, who felt they were insulated increasingly from their own physician. The delay in receiving a return call from the nurse after the secretary took the message earlier in the day was a further frustration. The size of our staff was becoming unwieldy as well as expensive. Something had to be done.

The solution was quite simple. A receptionist was retained to greet the patients, send their charts back to notify the doctor they were present, total their charge slips and collect their fees.

A telephone operator answers all lines promptly and refers the call directly to the nurse who works with that patient's own doctor. If it is a question about their bill or an insurance form, they are referred to one of the two computer operators who can supply this information. The telephone operator maintains a log of all calls, so each doctor–nurse team can be aware of their efficiency in answering calls and supplying sufficient patient information to keep return calls to a minimum.

Each doctor's own nurse takes all of his calls, obtains the necessary information, answers most questions herself, has the file librarian obtain the chart, makes appropriate appointments in her doctor's own appointment book, or records the information on a call slip which is later affixed permanently to the record after the physician has reviewed it and decided what action is required (see Figure 1). Since each nurse is working in her own doctor's particular 'corner' of the office, he is readily accessible himself to answer questions or occasionally talk to the patient. This ready access, direct to their own doctor, is much appreciated by the patients and is very efficient.

A medical assistant is assigned to each doctor. Ours are graduates of a two-year university course. They summon patients from the waiting room, place them in one of the three examining rooms allocated to each doctor, drape them, obtain their vital signs and record their complaint in the chart. They provide direct assistance to the physician as required for procedures such as pelvics or minor surgery. After the patient is seen by the doctor and he has recorded their prescriptions and instructions in the chart, the medical assistant copies prescriptions for the apothecary, gives injections and physical therapy, records electrocardiograms, and dispenses diets, patient instruction materials and any drugs prescribed from the office.

The nurse provides back-up to her medical assistant for any of the preceding, does venepunctures and performs basic in-office laboratory procedures. Return appointments also are her responsibility.

This physician–nurse–medical assistant team provides personal care for one physician's patients. It is our experience that by assigning one team to each physician, any number of family physicians could be housed in one facility and not deprive the patient of direct personal access to their own doctor.

When the doctor is out of the office, his nurse and medical assistant have time to perform interval Pap smears, do weight or blood pressure check-ups, interval baby checks and Denver development evaluations, and provide patient education for prenatals, hypertensives and diabetics. The doctor's telephone calls are answered by his nurse as usual, and emergency calls are referred by her to the other physicians in at the time, on a rotational basis.

Appointments

The efficient flow of any work day in the office is dependent upon the proper allocation of time to each patient. This probably is the most challenging system of any group practice, for many reasons. The hazards and unwieldy aspects of having appointments assigned at a front desk for a number of doctors with a limitless variety of patients, have already been noted in the preceding section. Ideally, each physician should have one or two staff people rotate the responsibility for his own appointment book.

DATE	TIME	CALLER		TEL. NOS.	
DR.	ALLERGIES	NAME OF PT.		AGE	TEMP.
MESSAGE					
R$_x$					APPT.

Figure 1   The call slip

Only in this manner can his own particular practice style be adhered to successfully. Even with such personal staff there will still be problems with patients who fail to describe their true problem over the phone for whatever reason. There will always be patients who complicate the appointment schedule by bringing along another member of the family to be checked, or those who will wish to have multiple symptom complaints attended to in addition to the one for which they were worked into the schedule. For these reasons, any appointment system must have some flexibility with catch-up time between segments.

We book patients into a four column appointment book. In the first column the advance booking for new patients and regular patient check-ups is allocated twenty minutes with the physician and restricted to one per hour. Two ten minute appointments for long term follow-ups on patients with chronic illness previously diagnosed, such as hypertension or diabetes, also are entered in the first column in each hour.

The second column is reserved for two short-term rechecks such as an acute middle ear infection or rash follow-up, and two quick checks for acute illnesses that have just occurred.

The third column is reserved for additional quick checks in a period where the office is overwhelmed with an epidemic of sore throats or gastroenteritis. Acute emergencies also are entered in the third column. When the necessity for a third column booking becomes apparent, the twenty minute appointment in the first column is rescheduled, thus opening up time to keep the schedule within bounds.

The fourth column is reserved to book time with our nurses for lab procedures, electrocardiograms, physical therapies, individual and group counselling, injections, and Denver development testing, much of which they can do when the physician is not in. Time is also set aside in this column for the preparation and testing of patients at the time of their visit with the physician. For example, new patients and complete physicals are booked with the nurse fifteen minutes before they see the physician. This provides time for the patient to complete a comprehensive history questionnaire, to familiarize themselves with our office policy brochure and to have their vital signs taken and be draped properly for examination.

Counselling sessions with the physician are scheduled outside the regular appointment schedule and usually are twenty minutes in duration.

In group practices, appointment schedules for all of the doctors should be arranged so that the office is covered by at least half of the group at all times, including vacation periods. Moreover, staggering hours enables us to cover the office from eight in the morning to six at night without imposing an inordinate number of hours on any one physician. Finally, this attention to scheduling permits each physician more efficiency by working with more examining rooms without acquiring additional office space. Ideally, each physician should have a minimum of three examining rooms at his disposal. With proper scheduling, four or five physicians can work efficiently in an office with only nine regular examining rooms.

Workload and personnel rostering

In a group practice there must be an overall master plan for scheduling all personnel and properly proportioning the workload. The basic decisions are the number of hours the office is to be open and the number of hours each physician wishes to work. The physician hours are then staggered to cover the office hours with as much depth as possible.

A basic business staff is assigned to cover the front office during all business hours. Every member of the business staff should be trained in the basic aspects of each job. This enables them to cover for each other daily to keep each individual's hours to a minimum. Also this insures coverage for vacations and illness. In our office the public must be met, the phone answered, and charts pulled. Our receptionist, telephone operator, file librarian, two computer operators, and the office manager assure a continuous operation of the three basics, ten hours a day, five days a week, and five hours on Saturday, without exceeding a forty hour week for anyone on a regular basis.

The same attention to rostering applies to the nursing staff. A nurse and a medical assistant must be in the office for each doctor scheduled. Since each doctor in our group averages less than twenty-eight hours a week in the office, there are ample hours for each doctor's nurse to be booked on her own and to attend to other nursing duties. The medical assistants can be rotated among the doctors so that three can cover four doctors in our office, for example, and still have time to help the nurses with their duties.

Work rosters must be worked out carefully for each office and posted. In addition, a large calendar for the year should be included on the business office bulletin board to post all vacation and meeting times for everyone to see and plan accordingly.

Communications

In Chapter 10 of this text, under 'General office equipment', a communication system is described for the individual office which can be expanded easily to a large group practice.

An adequate number of incoming telephone lines to accommodate calls cannot be emphasized too much in terms of communication with the public. Also there must be private lines unencumbered to permit outgoing calls. The telephone company will survey your needs and recommend proper equipment.

There should be some provision for answering calls to the office when the office is closed. Electronic equipment can be attached to the phone to answer, record messages, and play them back to the physician on call when he calls in. In metropolitan areas, an answering service can be obtained to cover the telephone and notify the physician on call. Many use a radio signal transmitted to a small receiver carried by the physician on his person.

Internal office communication can be achieved by adding telephone extensions equipped with intercom lines and speakers. This equipment can be leased from the telephone company, or private systems can be purchased from commercial sources and attached to the public telephone lines. A paging system can be incorporated into this system or installed separately. The larger the group, the greater the necessity for a sophisticated intra-office communication system.

Communication between the individual physician and the staff working with him can utilize the same paging system as the business office. However, in many offices a separate system is installed to facilitate the doctor–patient–nurse interaction.

One of these is a simple set of coloured flags mounted in the hall over each examining room doorway. Each colour can be assigned a different message, such as: patient waiting, doctor in room, nurse needed, nurse in room, or room clear.

A more elaborate communication system involving coloured lights is available. These can be activated on a panel in each examining room and displayed in the hall over each doorway and on a master panel in the nurses station.

Another helpful and very simple communication method is the use of coloured clothes pins attached to the charts when they are placed in the hallway pocket outside each examining room. These can advise the doctor of the type of appointment at a glance: clear denotes twenty minute appointment; green, a ten minute one; yellow, a recheck; and red, a quick check.

Other aspects of communication important to a group practice include those which promote staff interaction and cooperation. The posting of work rosters and the calendar of time off for the year, mentioned previously, promote adequate communication. In addition, there must be regular staff meetings to permit exchange of ideas and feelings. These include separate meetings of the business staff and the nursing staff and the physicians themselves. Intercommunication between these groups is accomplished through regular meetings of the business manager, head nurse and the physician in charge.

Group communication is a unique aspect of group practice in its potential for promoting individual growth. The expertise of each group is enhanced by regular exchange of ideas and experience. Secretaries, nurses and doctors alike are benefited.

Accounting

Posting charges by hand to an individual account card and daily logging of charges becomes quite cumbersome in a volume practice, and impossible in a large group practice. Therefore, it is necessary to utilize systems which expedite these accounting chores.

The simplest is a peg-board system which permits the simultaneous recording of charges and payments and balance due by superimposing the patient charge slip over a monthly statement and a master log sheet. The log sheet can be totalled at the end of the day to permit a day-to-day summary of productivity and accounts receivable. The patient account card can have up to three statements attached, one of which can be removed and mailed to the patient each month, or the account card itself can be photocopied or duplicated using the office duplicating equipment. This system is said to be practical in an office with eight hundred to a thousand charges per month.

Larger practice volume can be handled more efficiently by performing the above operations by an accounting machine available from a number of business machine manufacturers. The larger number of statements would require high speed copying equipment and, ideally, a machine to fold, stuff, seal and stamp statements for mailing. Volume up to fifteen hundred charges per month is ideal.

The accounting system most efficient for a large group practice is that handled by computer and described in detail in Chapter 10 of this text. A charge slip with a carbon copy is prepared for each patient to be seen and any outstanding balance obtained from the computer entered thereon. After the physician sees the patient, he has only to mark the printed code for the service rendered and enter the diagnosis or its code. The reception- ist enters the appropriate charge for each service and totals them. She records any payment received and the outstanding balance remaining, if any. The carbon is given to the patient providing him with an itemized account of services rendered, payment received, balance due, and diagno- sis. In most instances, patients can submit these copies to insurance carriers for payment, or keep them for tax purposes. The charge slips then go to a computer operator who enters the data on each patient.

An alternate system utilizes a charge card which can be marked by the physician and receptionist to record the patient visit transaction, and then scanned by the computer to enter the data and print out an itemized statement to hand to the patient while he or she is in the office.

In either event, the computer can be instructed to prepare statements on all patients with outstanding balances. These can either be printed in the office in a presealed envelope suitable for mailing, or in the form of open statements which can be folded, stuffed and sealed by hand or machine for mailing.

Finally, the computer is capable of providing productivity records on each physician and totals of charges and balances at any point in time for any period – day, month, and year-to-date.

Each of the systems described above – peg-board, accounting machine, and computer – is increasingly expensive in the order presented. However, with increased volume, each is cost-effective in its own right.

Data control

One of the greatest challenges to any medical group is the storage of data in such a form that it is easily retrieved and interpreted by any member of the group. This requires a charting system that furnishes basic information at a glance.

The patient's problems and medications can be entered on a flow sheet as illustrated in Figure 2. Allergies and important past history are noted in the margins. Another flow sheet contains immunizations and laboratory data (see Figure 3). These are kept in the front of the chart folder and provide an overall view of the patient in a minimum of time. Detailed information can be recorded on the progress sheets which are printed with a column for each system; if the individual physician wishes, a check-off system can be used here also.

All of this information can be committed to computer if this is available. If the patient is being seen on a regular appointment, a print-out of the last three visits is obtained, or at a minimum, the problem list and medication list.

It is mandatory in a group practice, where one doctor is covering for another, that there be absolute control of medications, specifically tracking of refill prescriptions.

The other major data problem in a group practice is telephone calls after hours as well as during office hours. Every telephone call message is recorded on a special form with adhesive backing which permits this to be

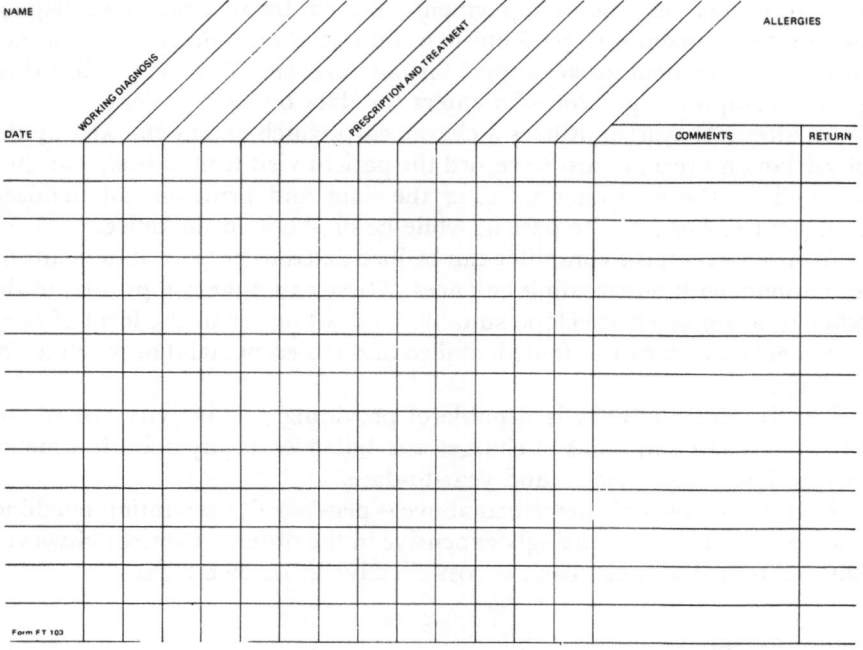

Figure 2   The flow sheet

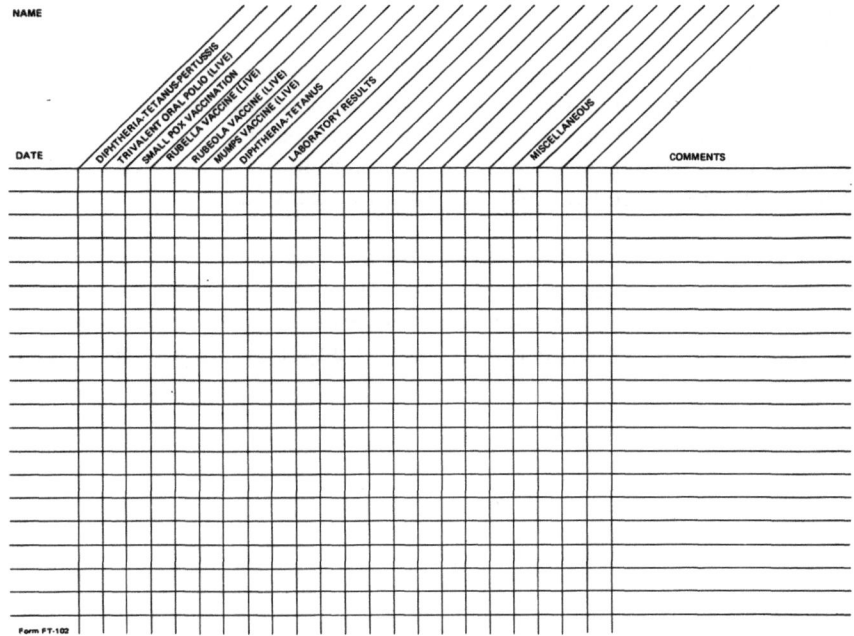

Figure 3   Flow sheet for immunizations and laboratory data

mounted ultimately in the patient's chart on the current progress sheet (see Figure 1). The group physician on call keeps a supply of these on hand to record the data on each patient contact. After the patient's own physician has had a chance to see the message the next day or whenever, it is then filed. These same forms are used for calls to the office also. Every patient contact with the office becomes a matter of record.

Stock control

One of the advantages of group practice is the savings realized by purchasing office and practice supplies in larger quantities. However, the control of such purchases can become a real problem. There are two major limitations: storage space and available funds. Both are obvious.

We try to spread our purchases over the entire year by preparing a budget for such purchases and requiring our office manager and head nurse to buy within these limits. The quantity of bulky items must be restricted to the storage space available. The quantity of perishable drugs is governed by the time of expected usage.

Each nurse and nurse assistant monitors a different aspect of supplies, maintaining a usage log. All orders for medical supplies are coordinated through the head nurse.

The front office supplies are the sole responsibility of the office manager, who has a separate budget for these.

Even sample drugs are assigned to a medical assistant in each area of the office. She is responsible for seeing that sample drugs are stored in an organized fashion, so that they can be retrieved easily.

Finally, the medical assistants are responsible for their own block of examining rooms to see that they are fully stocked with necessary supplies at all times.

The larger the group, the more complex the stock control problem becomes. The secret of control is the division of responsibility for different segments among all members of the staff, overall coordination through the office manager and the head nurse, and a budget to spread the expense over the entire year.

10

Facilities and Equipment in General Family Practice

B. LESLIE HUFFMAN JR. (USA)

Most of us who have practised family medicine for a few years have found ourselves in an acute medical situation at one time or another, equipped only with our own personal sensory and motor modalities. At such moments, we would have given anything for a few basic pieces of equipment, and even more for a well-equipped facility.

Except for such emergencies, few of us are inclined to appreciate fully the advantages of adequate, well-planned facilities and equipment. In fact, too often we take for granted our everyday office where we spend the majority of our practice lifetime. We allow our offices to grow with our practice and the needs of the day without careful planning in advance. The wastes and inefficiency incurred would more than match the cost of doing it the right way, not to mention the pleasure and daily satisfaction we receive as a bonus for our efforts in creating an efficient office environment.

I have designed and equipped three offices in my own family practice lifetime. In addition, I have had the opportunity to inspect a wide variety of family practices throughout the world. I have learned from them all. What I shall describe for you in this chapter, however, is not an amalgamation of what I have seen and learned, but a description of my own practice and the family practice teaching modules where I work. It would be unrealistic to believe that these can be replicated world-wide or even in all parts of my own country. However, I hope that you will find something in these pages which you can adapt to your own practice, and in the process improve the quality of your own everyday life.

OFFICE DESIGN

Whether you are practising in a cottage or an enormous office complex, space is a primary consideration. Basic design requirements are 92.9 square metres (one thousand square feet) per physician. This formula applies to multiple physician groups of any six practising full time. It does not take into account economies achieved by sharing space, staggering hours and free time. (This was covered in Chapter 9.)

Ideally, space should be located central to the practice served. In acquiring a new facility, the patients should be surveyed to assure its convenience to them. Access roads and public transportation are important considerations. Moreover, the location should provide adequate parking, grade access over curbs for wheelchairs and an elevator if the practice is not located on ground level.

Support facilities should be nearby, including pharmacy, X-ray, and laboratory. In more remote locations, some or all of these can be included in the family practice office itself.

Typical space allocation in a solo family practice is outlined in Table 1:

Table 1 *Space allocation in square metres* (92.9 square metres per family physician)

Reception area	16.7	Nurse station/laboratory	9.3
Business office	14.9	Consultation room	11.1
Examination room	8.4	Lavatory/toilet	2.3
Examination room	8.4	Common area/hall	10.7
Examination room	11.1		

The reception area should provide space for twice the number of patients seen in one hour. Assuming a maximum of seven patients an hour, seating should be provided for fourteen persons. 16.2 square metres (180 square feet) provides 1.16 square metres (12.85 square feet) per person which is quite adequate.

The business office must include filing space which is based on the number of patients. In practice, an area almost as large as the reception room will be required – 14.9 square metres (160 square feet) is suggested.

Examination rooms should be large enough for four persons and a comparable area for equipment. 8.4 square metres (90 square feet) is minimal and 9.3 square metres (100 square feet) is even better. One examination room should be larger to make room for therapeutic needs, which can be accommodated in a room with a curtain divider to facilitate dual usage. Over three linear metres of cabinets are combined in these rooms, providing in each room base cabinets with sinks mounted on laminated, stain-resistant surfaces, and wall mounted cabinets above.

The nurses station and laboratory combine comfortably into a 9.3 square metre area (100 square feet). This includes over three metres of base cabinets with a stainless steel sink, and again wall cabinets above.

The lavatory or toilet provides adequate space for a sink or vanity with a mirror above, and a water closet. Only 2.3 square metres (25 square feet) are needed.

A consultation room is a must for a family physician to see patients just for a talk and a good listen. Its size should be such that it appears uncrowded and uncluttered. Add space for the practice library, a work desk and comfortable chairs for the doctor and the patient. 11.1 square metres (120 square feet) should be roomy enough.

The common area and hall space is not a productive area at first glance. In fact, it may appear to be the most expensive of all, if poorly planned. However, space for patient and personnel flow is a necessity. Careful planning will keep it to a productive minimum. 10.7 square metres (115 square feet) should be more than enough for our basic practice unit.

Decor in all areas should be bright and cheerful. Use a lot of colour with tastefully selected accents just as you would in your own home. Avoid expensive, one-of-a-king displays which might be damaged or borrowed.

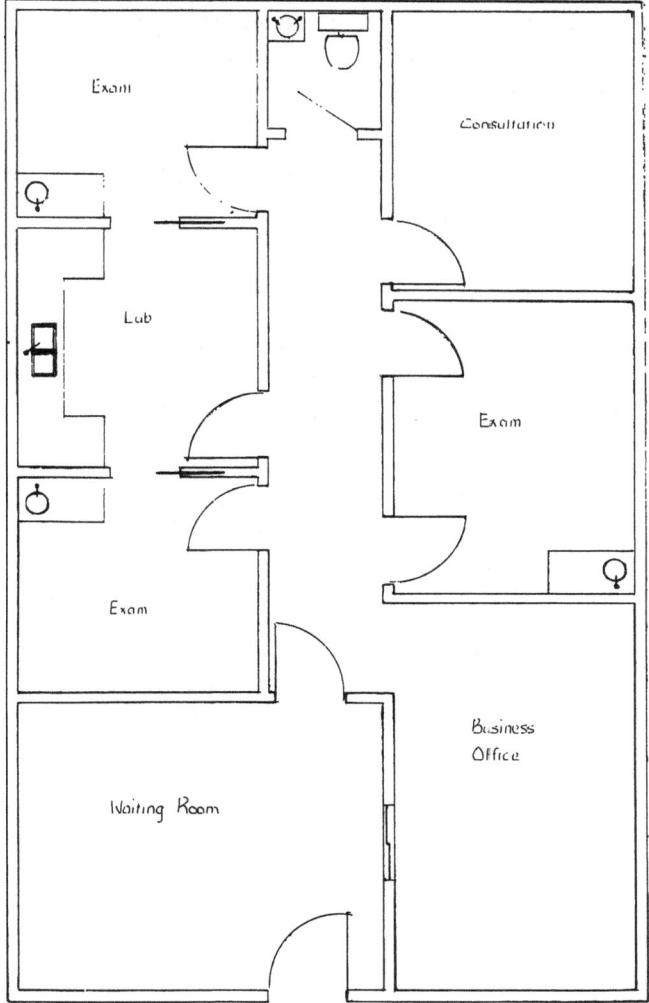

Figure 1   A family practice office (92.3 square metres)

A suggested design is illustrated which brings the above space allocations together in a very practical manner.

EQUIPMENT SELECTION

How a general/family practice office should be equipped depends greatly on its location – proximity to laboratory and X-ray services, availability of pharmacy, and access to hospital support facilities – and on the spectrum of the practice. My own practice is located in a medical complex containing all of the above support services, with a general hospital next door. Even under these circumstances, we perform some routine laboratory studies in the office. Most minor surgery also is done in our own 'operatory'. The primary reasons are convenience and lower cost to the patient. As far as the spectrum of the practice is concerned, ours is a full range from paediatrics to geriatrics, including obstetrics and minor surgery.

In purchasing office equipment, one should keep in mind the fact that most items are a one-time purchase and should last a practice lifetime. Therefore, it is wise to buy the best quality one can afford. I further rationalize this by telling my staff that our patients surely deserve the best.

General office equipment

Reception room. The basic furniture for any office should be comfortable and sturdy. Modular design furniture provides the most utility in the least space. Comfortable cushions and contoured seats make waiting time less distasteful.

Other ways to make the time pass faster and more constructively include a childrens' corner with a few basic indestructible toys and books. Adults appreciate current reading material consisting of magazines with short articles of general interest.

A bulletin board in the waiting area can keep patients posted on what is new in medicine, and stress major concerns such as immunization schedules and intervals for check-ups. Patient education is a must in order to make them partners in their own health care. In addition to bulletin boards, selected patient education pamphlets of general interest can be placed in the reception area. In some offices, audiovisual programmes are shown to the patients while they are waiting. Personally, I feel that these should be shown to patients on an individualized, selected basis, preferably in a separate patient education area or in the examination room itself. Audiovisuals can be videotapes displayed on a television monitor, or film cassettes shown on a portable projector. A wide variety of professionally produced audiovisuals are available for both modalities at the present time. Their growing popularity promises an infinite variety in the future at a reasonable cost.

Floor coverings throughout the office should be comfortable under foot and most durable in the reception and business areas, nursing station and operatory. Carpet is very satisfactory in most areas with today's durable weaves. However, tiles may be more practical in high soilage conditions.

If local weather necessitates, include adequate coat racks and storage for umbrellas and overshoes.

The reception area is the patient's introduction to your office. Make it a pleasant one.

Business office. Your receptionist is the patient's first personal contact. Her desk must be located in view of the patient waiting area, yet be readily accessible to record storage and nursing staff. I detest windows which block patients out entirely from the business office. This counter and desk area should be as open as possible. The counter should be at a comfortable cheque-writing height, and the desk area should be spacious and un-crowded. A typewriter is a must at this location, as well as access to all chart forms and disability and return to work forms, which will be completed here. An adding machine and a cash box will be a part of the front desk, while in larger group practices this function may be relegated to individual physician team areas. Toys or trinkets for younger patients may be dispensed from the front desk. Finally, the office communications system, internal and external, must be centred here.

Communication with the outside requires an adequate number of telephone lines to deal with the volume of calls. There should be a minimum of one listed outside line for each physician, plus an unlisted line for emergency in-coming calls and internal office use. If your patients experience too much difficulty in contacting your office, add outside lines on a rotary basis, so that if line one is busy, line two automatically will ring, and so on.

Some type of intercom is very helpful, either as part of the telephone system itself, or as a separate arrangement. The former is more versatile and compact; speakers can be incorporated into each extension phone for paging. Combination telephone – intercom systems can be leased from the telephone company or purchased from a number of manufacturers.

In my own family practice group, we have a combined system acquired through a lease–purchase arrangement that has a capacity for fourteen incoming lines and thirty-four extension phones. This permits an extension phone in every room and at every station. We have an unlisted line for personal calls and a direct line to the hospital next door, including all of its extensions.

Records have been discussed in Chapter 8 of this text. However, in discussing equipment and furnishings in this regard I would note my own preference for open shelf filing, which is the most accessible. If there are severe space limitations, revolving shelves in an electrically powered carousel will permit much greater storage capacity and still offer the advantages of open filing. The proper shelf is brought to the front operating level by pushing the correct button – truly a gadgeteer's delight.

The business office needs a copying machine which is fast and makes good, legible copies. There is a wide variety of these from which to select.

Buy the best you can afford, to avoid frequent breakdowns and an illegible product.

Computer capabilities are being introduced into many practices today. I will discuss this in detail later. However, if this is in the future for your practice, the business office will have to accommodate at least a computer console and a printer.

Comfortable secretarial chairs are a must in every business office. Miscellaneous items include a postage meter and scales, staplers and staple removers, adequate files for all business forms and patient handouts, and a supply of stationery. A wide variety of patient education materials can be displayed in a large rack at the front desk to make these most accessible and useful. If more than one person consistently requires the use of a typewriter, it is more efficient to add a second machine to the business office. A list of minutiae would not be complete without Scotch tape, pre-inked rubber stamps for commonly written messages, a variable date stamp, and a cheque endorsement stamp. If the number of employees warrants the expense, you can save a great deal of confusion over hours worked by adding a time clock.

A real time-saver is dictating equipment which can be used to transcribe all business correspondence and patient data as well. Small hand-sized units are the most portable for recording; desk models have the advantage of being on-line to transcription equipment. In some areas, dictation can be done by telephone to an outside transcription service. In our own group, with adequate secretarial help, we prefer the small, hand-held units and transcription in-house.

Diagnostic equipment

Simplistic as it may seem, the basic diagnostic equipment in a family practice office is that which is contained within the physician himself or herself and carried on his or her person. My stethoscope, pen-light, tongue depressors, neurotome, pocket rule and bandage scissors are part of my attire; I would feel naked without them.

It is most efficient for each examining room to be equipped identically. The basic needs are: an examining table, scales for height and weight, a sphygmomanometer or aneroid for blood pressure, an otoscope and ophthalmoscope, vaginal specula and an anoscope, with an adequate light source for each. Tongue depressors, drape sheets and tissues complete the common supplies. Standard or electronic thermometers should be added to each room. A pillow for the examining table is a thoughtful addition.

Some comments on the basics. Electrically operated hi-lo examining tables certainly spare one's back and improve the view, and are easier for patients to mount, but they are expensive. One table, in addition to vertical manoeuverability, should have the hydraulics to incline forward for sigmoidoscopy. At least one paediatric examining table with built-in scales should be included. It is most functional to have both an adult examining table and a paediatric table in the same room to check mother and infant. Extra paediatric scales in another area adds versatility. The most accurate scales are beam balance. A mercury column is the most reliable and reproducible for blood pressure. Be careful to use the proper size arm cuff; every office should have one extra-large size and a paediatric size. Otoscopes and ophthalmoscopes should be continuously powered or have constant-charge power handles; no one should be diagnosing in the dark. You can use a light source and head mirror with stainless steel reusable vaginal speculae or disposable plastic ones. We use disposable ones with a built-in fibre-optic light source. The same applies to the anoscope.

Other diagnostic equipment does not have to be available in every room, but can be stored in special areas, such as the multiple-purpose examining room. Such equipment should include a tonometer to screen for glaucoma routinely in patients over forty years of age, an office spirometer to measure pulmonary function, a laryngeal mirror which may or may not have its own light source, nasal speculae, a sinus light, and a proctosigmoidoscope which can be a disposable fibre-optic lighted unit, using the same light source as the disposable vaginal speculum. Trays for catheterization and lumbar puncture also are on the disposable list, as well as gastric specimen sets.

Provision for electrocardiography is a necessity and can be accomplished in a variety of fashions. Basic recording equipment can be purchased to produce an electrocardiogram that can be mounted by the staff and interpreted by the physician. In some areas, recording equipment can be leased which will transmit the electrocardiogram by phone line to a computer centre which can provide a copy by return mail with interpretation; emergency readings are obtained by phone. In my own office, we have a computer terminal linked by phone line to the computer in our local hospital. When attached to the patient, a twelve lead electrocardiogram is recorded simultaneously in the office and the hospital, providing a copy in the office with interpretation by the computer, in a matter of minutes. An over-read by the cardiologist at the hospital can be obtained if desired on an individual basis. Stress testing can be done in the office by adding a bicycle or treadmill with monitoring equipment. The computer technology and stress testing equipment are relatively expensive and impractical for a solo family practice unless there is an unusual volume of patient application.

Office laboratory studies are a convenience for the doctor and an economy for the patient in regard to several basic tests. Our own minimum list includes the following:

Haemoglobin	Throat culture
WBC and differential	Urine culture with colony count
Blood sugar	Vaginal culture
Cholesterol	GC culture
Blood urea nitrogen	Mono spot test

Uric acid　　　　　　　　　　Pregnancy test
Triglycerides　　　　　　　　RA spot test
Prothrombin time　　　　　　Sedimentation rate
Haematocrit　　　　　　　　　Haemoccult.

The equipment for all the above requires a minimum of laboratory space. The tests can be performed accurately by regular office personnel; however, there should be provision for quality control by an outside laboratory.

Basic equipment includes a microscope, timer, urine test tapes (for sugar, albumen, blood, bile, acetone and urobilinogen) and a hygrometer. A number of manufacturers produce office colorimeters to do haemoglobin, blood sugar, cholesterol, uric acid, and blood urea nitrogen estimations. A more sophisticated version of this unit can produce its own SMA 12, and a similar unit permits prothrombin time determinations. A Wintrobe tube and pipette is all you need for measuring the sedimentation rate; add a centrifuge and you have a haematocrit. An office incubator with a CO_2 chamber and the appropriate culture media permit a wide variety of office cultures. Special office kits are available to test for pregnancy, rheumatoid arthritis, infectious mononucleosis, triglycerides, and occult blood. Digital read-out counters are available for blood counts. Gram staining equipment is a practical and simple addition when trained personnel are available. Potassium hydroxide is needed for fungus studies.

There are a number of additional tests that one can include if time and personnel and sufficient utilization justify the expense. For example, thyroid function can be measured, with office determination of T3, T4, and T7. With current technology the list of possibilities is almost limitless. One must take a practical look at his or her own situation and equip accordingly.

Office laboratory procedures can be expanded if there is not a commercial laboratory to which patients can be referred or to which specimens can be mailed for analysis. In these instances, a registered laboratory technician should be added to the staff and the equipment list expanded far beyond that required for the ordinary family practice office.

A number of years ago it was quite common to have a fluoroscope in the office and many had X-ray equipment for fractures of extremities and chest X-rays. This is very uncommon today if a full service radiological office is located nearby. If not, a small unit for emergency extremity films and chests can be purchased or leased. The manufacturers will provide detailed specifications for any necessary shielding. Automatic film processing equipment also is available for office use. This expenditure for space and equipment is justified only if the family practice is located at some distance from a professional X-ray office.

Therapeutic equipment

Nurses' station. The centre for office therapeutics is the nurses' station which must be located conveniently to the examining rooms and be equipped with a stainless steel sink, adequate cabinets for injectables and drugs dispensed, and refrigerated space.

The injectables which my associates and I employ are listed here for your information. Our individual preferences require some increased variety. The list is not intended to be comprehensive or all-inclusive.

Bacteriostatic water
Lidocain hydrochloride 1%
Bicillin LA 1 200 000 U tubex
Bicillin CR 900/300 U tubex
Bicillin CR 1 200 000 U tubex
Bicillin CR 600 000 U tubex
Penicillin G Procaine 300 000 U/ml
Penicillin G Procaine 2 400 000 U tubex and
Probenecid 0.5 g, 2 tablets
Oxytetracycline 50 mg/ml
Lincomycin hydrochloride monohydrate 300 mg/ml
Diphtheria and Tetanus toxoids with Pertussis vaccine, combined
Diphtheria and Tetanus toxoids combined (paediatric)
Tetanus toxoid
Tetanus and Diphtheria toxoids combined (adult)
Pneumococcal vaccine
Measles, mumps and rubella vaccine
Rubella vaccine
Mumps vaccine
Rubeola vaccine
Measles and rubella virus vaccine
Rubella and mumps vaccine
Influenza virus vaccine
Cholera vaccine
Tuberculin, old (Tine)
Poison ivy extract
Triamcinolone acetonide
Methyl prednisolone acetate
Dexamethasone 4 mg/ml
Dexamethasone-LA 8 mg/ml
Adrenocorticotrophic hormone, repository 40 U/ml
Epinephrine 1 mg/ml
Aminophyllin 250 mg/ml
Gammaglobulin
Testosterone cypionate 200 mg/ml
Estradiol cypionate 5 mg/ml
Testosterone enanthate 90 mg/ml and oestradiol valerate 4 mg/ml combined
Medroxyprogesterone acetate suspension 100 mg/ml

Propantheline bromide 15 mg/ml
Diclomine hydrochloride 10 mg/ml
Dimenhydrinate 50 mg/ml
Trimethobenzamide 100 mg/ml
Diazepam 5 mg/ml
Promethazine hydrochloride 50 mg/ml
Hydroxyzine hydrochloride 50 mg/ml
Morphine sulphate 15 mg/ml
Meperidine hydrochloride 50 mg/ml
Pentazocine lactate 30 mg/ml
Diphenhydramine hydrochloride 50 mg/ml
Furosemide 10 mg/ml
Mercaptomerin sodium 125 mg/ml
Cyanocobalamin 1000 mcg/ml
Phytonadione 10 mg/ml
Carbazochrome salicylate
Iron dextran injection 50 mg/ml
Gold sodium thiomalate 50 mg/ml
Aquasol A 15 mg or 50 000 U/ml
Kutapressin injection
Calcium gluconate 100 mg/ml.

It is not our practice to dispense drugs on any major scale, since we have a full service pharmacy or apothecary in our clinic building. However, we do stock a few basic drugs for the convenience of patients.

Potassium penicillin G 400 000 U
Tetracycline 250 mg
Nitrofurazone ointment
Mafenide acetate cream
Hydrocortisone cream 1%
Phenobarbital 30 mg
Meprobamate 400 mg
Aspirin compound
Prenatal vitamin
Vitamin B_{12} 25 mg
Prednisone 5 mg
Conjugated oestrogen 1.25 mg
Norethindrone acetate and ethinyloestradiol
Oxytocin citrate buccal 200 units.

Common drugs stocked for office treatments and occasionally dispensed include Cantharidin collodion and 25% podophyllin in tincture benzoin. Oral polio vaccine, trivalent, is dispensed from disposable pipettes.

Moreover, we have organized storage space for samples to make them easily available for starter doses and for total therapy of needful patients.

Disposable syringes and needles are very inexpensive today, especially when we consider the expense of sterilization and the risks of contamination. We stock mostly 2 ml syringes, plus a few 5 ml and 10 ml sizes. Needle assortment includes 18, 21, 23 and 25 gauge. Alcohol pledgets are individually sealed in foil. Velcro tourniquets are available for venepuncture.

Drugs for emergency use should be kept in a separate container. Our emergency tray contains the following:

Disposable needles: 19 (1)   21(3)   23   (3)
Disposable syringes: 3 ml/25 needle (1)
                      3 ml/21 needle (2)
                      3 ml/23 needle (2)
                      5 ml/23 needle (1)
                      10 ml/23 needle (1)
Lidocaine hydrochloride 100 mg (20 mg/ml) in a pre-filled syringe
Hydrocortisone sodium succinate (Mix-O-Vial) 100 mg and 250 mg
Epinephrine 1:1000, 30 ml vial
Nikethamide NF 25% 2 ml ampoule
Caffeine and sodium benzoate 0.5 g/2 ml ampoule
Deslanoside 2 ml ampoule
Aminophyllin 500 mg/2 ml ampoule
Aminophyllin 250 mg/10 ml ampoule
Hydroxyzine hydrochloride 100 mg/2 ml ampoule
Diphenhydramine hydrochloride 50 mg/1 ml ampoule
Adrenosem salicylate 2 ml ampoule
Conjugated oestrogens 25 mg i.v. pack
Promethazine hydrochloride 50 mg/1 ml ampoule
Ethylnorepinephrine hydrochloride 2 mg/1 ml ampoule
Diazepam 5 mg/ml, 10 ml vial
Morphine sulphate 15 mg/ml, 30 ml vial
Meperidine hydrochloride 50 mg/ml, 50 ml vial
Alcohol pledgets (10).

In addition to the emergency drugs, every family practice office should have emergency resuscitation equipment. The minimum is an assortment of airways and a face mask with attached bag which can be compressed manually. A simple mechanical suction unit and canisters of oxygen with mask and tubing complete the emergency equipment. It is mandatory that all office personnel be familiar with this equipment; preferably all should be trained in cardiopulmonary resuscitation.

A very useful tray is one equipped for eye injuries. This should contain a topical anaesthetic such as benoxinate HCl, sodium fluorescein strips for staining, an ophthalmic irrigating solution, a cobalt blue light, a spud to remove foreign bodies from the cornea, an antibiotic for ophthalmic use, eye patches and Scotch tape. Our tray includes atropine sulphate 1% solution and dexamethasone sodium phosphate, 0.1% ophthalmic.

Another commonly used tray is one for cerumenosis. It contains a small basin and an ear syringe, plus a plastic drape that fastens around the neck, and a kidney basin to keep the rest of the patient dry. A new development is the adaptation of the water pick to replace the ear syringe; this delivers a pulsating stream of water to the external auditory canal and is far more effective.

Operatory. One examination room should be equipped as an operatory for minor office surgery. A small autoclave is necessary to sterilize instruments. The following sets should be available:

Excision set: Mayo dissecting scissors, straight; thumb tissue forceps; haemostatic forceps, straight (2); combination needle holder-scissors; Allis tissue forceps (2).

IUD set: Cervical tenaculum forceps; uterine sound; sponge forceps; uterine dressing forceps; long straight scissors.

Other instruments:

Small comedome extractor
Large comedome extractor
Foreign body extractor
Splinter forceps
Small suture removal set with sharp pointed scissors
Cervical biopsy forceps
Skin punch biopsy
Haemorrhoid forceps
Anal speculum
Toe-nail clipper
Tongue retractor
10 ml finger-tip control syringe
20 ml glass syringe.

No operatory would be complete without a safety razor with disposable blades. Another useful device is a battery-powered nail drill.

A good operating light is a must, as well as an examining table that will adapt to multiple positions such as are required for sigmoidoscopy. The operatory should be equipped with an electrocautery unit which can deliver both cutting and coagulating current to a variety of applicators, the most useful of which are the needle and wire loop. Many family physicians prefer a cryosurgical unit to the electric cautery even though they are more expensive. However, with good office utilization they are cost-effective.

The minutiae of a typical surgery includes vaseline gauze, iodoform gauze and rubber tubing for drains, and a fluoremethane combination in an aerosol. Our suture assortment lists 5-0 nylon, 4-0 nylon and chromic, 3-0 chromic and silk and gut – all with swaged needles in individual autoclaved packages. Disposable scalpels with both #11 and #15 blades are very practical. Surgical dressings include an assortment of Band Aids, 3 × 3 sterile gauze and Telfa pads, and Kerlex and adhesive tape rolls in a variety of widths. Disposable sterile gloves and bandage scissors complete this list.

For orthopaedic therapy our operatory is equipped with an assortment of aluminium splints that are padded and can be moulded easily. A quick-setting plaster is available in two-inch, three-inch and four-inch rolls. Elastic roll dressings in similar widths are stocked, as well as Webril padding. Roll gauze saturated with unna paste is very useful. Other supplies include an assortment of rubber heels for walking casts, child and adult crutches, stockinette in assorted widths, slings, clavicle splints, and cervical collars.

Newer cast materials are available in some areas that are moisture resistant. If there is sufficient volume of cast work, fibreglass type rolls are available which are porous and can be moulded and fixed under special lights. After proper application they can be immersed in water to permit bathing and swimming. This set-up is more expensive and not practical for our present volume.

Other cast supplies include disposable hot and cold packs, a cast spreader, an electric cast cutter, cast cutting scissors, and a ring cutter.

Plastic forearm and wrist splints, and aluminium posterior tibia and fibula knee length splints in assorted sizes are most useful.

Included in the operatory or similar ancillary area should be physical therapy. An elementary approach is practical in the office setting if one has adequate, well-trained staff. More involved manipulative therapy and prolonged rehabilitative therapy in our situation is best referred to our full service physical therapy department located elsewhere in the clinic. If this were not available to us, we could expand the in-house capabilities easily in order to fulfil this need.

Our basic equipment includes:

Hydrocollator Master   Unit (Model E-1) 1000 watts
Hydrocollator Steam Packs, Standard size (3), Neck contour (1)
Ultrasound and EMS (Rich-Mar   Corporation Model Delta-330)
Rich-Mar Lotion (water soluble and greaseless)
Wood physical therapy table with comfortable padding and
adequate pillows.

Examination rooms. The basic therapeutic modalities should be included in each examining room and should be located in the same place. In our office, the large operatory which can be used as an examining room has the same basic built-in cabinet for examining equipment as all our other examining rooms contain. Certainly, there is additional cabinet space for cast supplies and surgical equipment, but the basic unit is the same.

Each counter top includes sink with soap and paper towel dispensers, an otoscope and ophthalmoscope in a continuous charging base and an extension telephone. Cabinets above contain extra paper towels and disposable tissues and examining gloves, pillow, plastic emesis basin and round basin, hydrogen peroxide, and cytology supplies including glass slides, large Q-tips, endocervical pipettes and 5 ml syringe, fixative and acetic acid, and a naso-pharyngeal wire. Aerosols of topical anaesthetic, lubricant, and Betadine complete the upper cabinets.

The top drawer contains tongue depressors, alcohol and Betadine pledgets, K-Y Jelly, disposable gloves, silver nitrate applicators, two sizes of disposable ear specula for the otoscope, a nasal speculum, laryngeal and sinus light attachments for the otoscope, ear wicks, note pads for instructions and office policy hand-outs.

The second drawer is equipped with dressings including Telfa and sterile gauze pads, assorted widths of adhesive tape, paper tape, Kerlex, Band Aids and sterile paper strips for wound closure, cast scissors and bandage scissors, Q-tips, disposable scalpel with #11 and #15 blades, and disposable suture removal sets.

The lower drawer contains sanitary napkins, paper chest drapes and full length paper gowns.

Drawers in the end of the examining table contain disposable fibre-optic vaginal speculae and the transformer light source, cotton balls and large cotton-tipped applicators, anal speculae, and ring forceps.

Side drawers in the examining tables store disposable paper tissues and personal cleansing wipes, plus additional paper drapes.

COMPUTERS IN OFFICE PRACTICE

Today we live in the computer age. Information on the vast majority of the population of our world has been stored and can be retrieved through computer technology.

In our own area, computer adaptation to everyday family practice was begun in the 1960s. At that time, our local banks had computer time which could be rented to handle billing procedures for any business, including the practice of medicine. Tapes could be punched with the necessary information and mailed to computer centres for processing. Basic financial data could be accumulated such as accounts receivable and productivity, and statements for services rendered could be prepared and mailed.

The first major improvement in these basic services came in the late 1960s when computer banks were programmed especially for medical practice needs and made available to individual practices by installing computer terminals in the office, connected to the remote computer centres by phone line. Confidentiality was maintained by assigning access codes known only to the individual office and using separate frequencies on shared intercity phone lines. The almost limitless capacity of such a computer centre expanded the scope of data storage and retrieval such that all the records of a family practice could be computerized. Not only financial data, but also patient data could be included to whatever extent desired. My own family practice and most of our family practice residency teaching modules in this area subscribe to such a service.

In the 1970s minicomputers were developed which today permit one to purchase or lease a totally in-house operation. This circumvents to some extent the problems of down time and sometimes slow response that plagues on-line computers. However, the capacity and versatility of programming available is limited. In-house computers also are subject to down time and the problems of local service.

Cost is a major determinant in the type of computer service elected and the extent to which it is utilized. Basic financial services can be obtained at a cost equivalent to one secretary, as a general rule, from an outside computer service. An in-house computer will cost about the same as two secretaries, but will provide more versatility. The widest range of services currently is available from an on-line computer centre, but will cost about as much as three secretaries. Obviously, the larger the group and/or the volume of the practice, the more computer technology one can utilize on a practical basis.

My own four family physician group is on-line to a computer centre especially programmed to serve some two thousand family physicians in northern Ohio. We have two computer terminals in our office – one in the front business office to access data and another in the back to which data is fed throughout the practice day. Also, at the front is a high speed printer which will produce a copy of the data displayed on the screen of the terminal in a matter of seconds.

The five basic applications of the computer in office practice are the storage and retrieval of financial data, health data, practice research, patient education, and physician education.

Financial data

As stated previously, the most basic utilization and the earliest application of computers to medical practice was for storage and retrieval of financial information.

Basic data required is the patient's name, family member responsible, address, and outstanding balance. Illustrated is our basic data screen. Itemized charges are fed to the computer by tape or on-line daily to enable the physician to monitor his daily or monthly or annual productivity and to analyse the scope of practice. Entering daily receipts permits the computer to prepare itemized statements for the patients which can be printed and mailed outside the office if one is willing to pay for this extra service. With this additional information the computer is able to track and age accounts receivable. The addition of a diagnosis for each patient visit

```
     365        BERNARD LESLIE HUFFMAN JR        ADM RECORD    SEC  1*
STREET DEEPWATER FARM                * CITY GRAND RAPIDS           *
STATE :OHIO                 *ZIP 43522*SOC SEC. :413-48-0784      *
BIRTHDATE 02/24/29 *HEIGHT :68   *WEIGHT 160  *NOTE1:          *
HOME PHONE 832-5445*BUS  PHONE :893-2321*EXT. ·     *NOTE2 MD  *ACC:   *
INS. B/C B/S          * CONTRACT #:572192      * PLAN CODE ·        *
SERV CODE :           *GROUP #:31120    *MEDICARE #:           * SEX M*
C/O:                                                                   *
BILL TO SAME                        *
```

Figure 2   Basic computer data screen

makes it possible for the computer to complete the necessary insurance forms. At this point in time, most of the practices on computer confine their usage to preparation of statements, analysis of the practice and productivity, tracking accounts receivable, and printing insurance forms.

Information on payables can be included in order to have the computer prepare cheques to pay monthly expenses and the payroll for employees. Each individual physician can have a special access code known only to the physician and perhaps the spouse and/or the accountant, behind which can be stored data on personal finances. Thus the computer can log monthly bills for the individual and balance the cheque book as well.

The financial data capabilities can be managed quite well by an in-house minicomputer or by transmitting data by tape or phone to an outside centre. Utilization to this extent should be within range of practical expense for any busy small group practice or a very large solo practice.

Health data

A high capacity on-line or in-house system can contain a complete patient data base, to which can be added visit data organized in a problem-oriented fashion. Any patient information can be displayed in a flow chart to provide sequential data on blood pressure, weight, immunizations, laboratory or roentgenological findings. The appointment system, itself, can be entered into the computer and be utilized to recall patients for necessary preventive care such as periodic examination and immunizations. High risk population groups can be singled out by the computer and summoned to receive special treatment when current medical knowledge demands such care.

Practice research

Up to now most medical research has been conducted on inpatients and university medical centre clinic populations which represent only about two percent of the medical care in the world. The ninety-eight percent seen in the community ambulatory care facilities has not been researched to any great extent.

The challenge is to identify early disease in population groups in our practices and to research their outcome data in the practice setting. A future use of the computer in office practice will be to identify, for example, our diabetics and our hypertensives, and to document their therapy and response. The potential for practice research is limitless; the computer is an essential facilitator in this regard.

Patient education

Another potential application of computer technology to office practice is its ability to test patient's knowledge of their health and disease, and to furnish them with new information about themselves. A number of our computer programming centres currently are in the process of developing such programmes.

Physician education

Finally another future use of the computer will be in the area of physician education. For example, patient management problems can be presented to the physician on the computer terminal screen with multiple branching, allowing the physician to explore current knowledge and acquire new data in complete privacy.

Another current example of the use of the computer in education is the preparation of in-training assessment examinations, and certifying and recertifying examinations from question items stored for this purpose. An adaptation of this would be individually designed tests on one or more selected subjects presented to the physician in the office on his or her own computer terminal.

Recommended reading

Brandejs, J.F. and Huffman, B.L. Jr. (1984). The Use of Computers in Practice. In Rakel, R.E. (ed.) *Textbook of Family Practice*. Third edn. Chapter 69. (Philadelphia: W.B. Saunders)

Huffman, B.L. Jr. (1984). Appointment Scheduling. *ibid*

Godkin, M.A. and Catlin, R.J.D. (1984). Office Design, chapter 70. *ibid*

11
Applied Research in General Family Practice

JOSEPH LEVENSTEIN (SOUTH AFRICA)

General family practice in its brief history as a 'new' discipline has not devoted a major part of its academic effort to the area of research. If we understand research as being directed to the discovering of new knowledge, consolidating or verifying observations, or merely the chronicling and analysing day-to-day events, the area to be covered is vast. Many difficulties have been encountered in the planning and execution of this research. The most important problems have been related to the fact that in this stage of the discipline's infancy, all are not agreed about what general practice is, and also while many have been at pains to describe the differences between episodic hospital based care and continuing ambulatory general practice care, the hospital based model has been the one that often has been used as the research model in general practice. Thus many have been 'frightened off' research, and much still remains unwritten and unresearched. Another possible reason for the research effort being of such low priority is the fact that with limited personnel, much of the academic activity has been directed to the formulation of undergraduate courses, vocational training schemes, and administration generally. It is hoped that this brief review of opportunities may stimulate some to initiate research, or a desire to participate in research. To participate in research, you don't necessarily have to set up an original hypothesis to be tested or even design a trial, you can be just one of the participants.

Those that have attempted research have been imaginative and informative, in many instances opening several areas of study, not only for general practice, but for other medical disciplines. This chapter is written from a personal viewpoint and represents the experience of a general practitioner in full time practice, and thus indicates the opportunities available for the practising doctor if he is able to discipline himself, overcome his negative attitudes to research, and regard his practice as a research laboratory.

Research can be directed to several areas:

1. Content of general practice – epidemiology, natural history of disease.

2. Management interventions
3. Relationship of doctor and patient – the effects their attitudes have on illness and its outcome
4. Process of consultation
5. The practice itself and its organization
6. Doctors' educational process
7. Patients' educational process
8. A comparison between different primary health care systems
9. Effect of primary health care on health problems.

A general practitioner initiating research can do so *individually*, or as part of a group – *collaborative* study. In so doing, he must not hesitate to use expertise from other disciplines where it is appropriate. He must however, be mindful to use this advice as an adjuvant to his research and not allow the priorities of another discipline to interfere with his legitimate study.

If a general practitioner wishes to embark on a project, he must be careful to define exactly what he is setting out to do. For example, he may have noted that patients of a particular occupation are more likely to become hypertensive, or that 90% of his out of hours work comes from a small group of his patients. What does he now need to validate these observations? Firstly, he must be an accurate observer, have appropriate notes, and have a ready means of identifying his patients from his files. Ideally he has a practice age-sex register and knows his practice population at risk. He can now decide that he has enough data to do a study – to analyse the outcomes of patients he has already seen (*retrospective study*), or alternatively do a *prospective study* analysing clearly looked for data according to a protocol. Prospective studies have inevitably more reliability and validity, and data can be uniformly collected.

DRAWING UP A SIMPLE TRIAL

Let us say the following *hypothesis* is to be investigated: 'Lorry drivers are more likely to develop hypertension'. The general practitioner has noted that 10 of his 12 patients that have this occupation are found to be 'hypertensive' (he must have already defined what he means by hypertension and the methodology used in diagnosing this hypertension). He may then be satisfied in recording this observation as it is. However, he may wish to seek *controls* within his own practice to compare the incidence of hypertension in people with different occupations. He obtains files from other patients of the same sex and age and compares them with those of his study group in areas such as similar length of service at a particular occupation, other illnesses, and so on. He then finds an incidence, for example, of 3 hypertensives out of 12 in his matched controls (who are clerks, for example). Now he takes his work to a statistician who tells him whether his results are *statistically significant* or not, that is, could they have just occurred by chance, or is the finding significant? He now seeks reference material and advice about his findings for his *review* on the subject. Finally, he states his *findings* and makes his *conclusions*, for example, 'lorry drivers are more susceptible than a control group of clerks to hypertension at a statistically significant level'. However, the statistician may say the numbers are too few for any meaningful observation, so he may want to involve other colleagues in a joint venture to achieve significant results. He may also postulate further areas for research, such as that hypertension is brought on by stress. This is straightforward research by any standards and well within the compass of any general practitioner.

The doctor has demonstrated all the features needed for research – an alert, original mind, the discipline to follow an idea through, and the creation of protocols which can receive data obtainable in general practice. This is in fact all that is needed. Assistance is always available to help with methodology, statistics and bibliography.

THE CONTENT OF GENERAL PRACTICE

The content of general practice is unique and probably represents the most important area for research. Firstly, there are the diseases that are supposedly well documented, but which can present in many and as yet unrecorded fashions. Then there are the diseases that are seen only by primary care physicians, and finally there are the many undifferentiated symptoms which require careful description of their natural histories.

Pioneer work has been done by such as Hodgkin and Fry in defining the problems of practice. These pioneers have noted disease patterns occurring in general practice and have compared them with hospital disease patterns, as well as looking at the natural histories of many commonly occurring conditions. I believe this type of work represents the beginnings of the rewriting of medicine. Knowledge of disease thus far, and consequently therapeutic interventions in these diseases, have all their origins rooted in observations from hospital based episodic doctors. It is extremely difficult to talk about the natural history of coronary heart disease, for example, which has a natural history of 40 years, if the only time one is treating it or observing it, is during a major complication such as myocardial infarction, which warrants hospitalization for only two weeks, let us say. Also there is that vast body of knowledge known only to general practitioners which must be chronicled. The natural histories of common and undifferentiated symptoms such as headache and tiredness, for example, all require careful observation of their nature, outcome and frequency. One of the major problems encountered in this approach has been our desire to use diagnoses or international disease classifications as a basis for our content, as opposed to problems as they really present.

Thus a general practitioner can contribute much to the knowledge of disease process, patient behaviour, family effects on illness and so on, merely by recording and observing. Examples are Addison's disease, which was first recorded in a few cases by careful observation, and James McKenzie's continuous chronicling of the natural history of heart disease.

I have been impressed by the factors that have precipitated hypertension in patients that have been normotensive all the while. Precipitating factors have included major stress events, viral infections and the onset of severe depression. These observations have been carefully documented and have been presented as hypotheses for possible further study.

A further example, in the behavioural field, is what flows from a consultation where a patient states 'I have just come for a check-up'! By carefully creating offers for patients, the majority of these patients reveal an underlying fear or psychological problem. Observations such as these are important in defining the content of general practice. For example, is this entered in a morbidity study as 'routine check-up' or as 'anxiety arising from father's recent myocardial infarction' or 'unresolved guilt associated with the death of that father', or all three!

I must issue one word of warning about this type of 'observational research'. It must purport to be what it is, and one must be very careful not to become anecdotal. The documentation must be complete, and observation should be over a long period. The observer must also realize that at the end he may be, at best, putting up a hypothesis for testing.

MANAGEMENT INTERVENTIONS

It is difficult to observe disease without relating it to *management*. Management in general practice covers a whole host of interventions from just observation (using time as a diagnostic and therapeutic tool) to active intervention or referral. To look at the commonest form of intervention, namely drug administration, have you ever stopped to consider how few trials of drugs, which are for use in ambulatory patients, are actually done in the community? Nearly all major drug trials on antihypertensive, musculoskeletal, antidiabetic, sedative and antidepressant drugs are performed in hospitals. The right place for these trials is surely in the area where the drugs are to be used – the community, and general practitioners are the ones to carry them out.

The South African general practitioner group has laid down rigid criteria for the acceptance of such trials. These include the usual ethical criteria, a strict scientific protocol, and the proviso that the trial will in no way be 'promotional'. Thus the type of trial they are prepared to carry out is often a 'world first' of a drug which is to be used in ambulatory practice. It is possible to conduct a therapeutic trial on your own, for example if one finds, maybe serendipitously, a new action of a drug already in use. In all cases, one should follow scientific and ethical procedures, seeking help and advice where appropriate.

An overall *'management intervention'* project to illustrate the role and value of general practitioners in medical care, is another fruitful area for research. The Cape GP Coronary Care Project, where 129 general practitioners collaborated over a 14 month period achieved its objective in showing 'that the general practitioner, having been educated as to the early prehospital management of acute myocardial infarction, could approximate the management effected by a mobile intensive coronary care unit'. Again, a management intervention can be carried out on one's own. A study to evaluate the possibility of predicting or preventing acute heart attacks by a vigorous approach to unstable angina, has recently been completed in my practice. I believe a major collaborative study would be needed to substantiate the initial findings.

DOCTOR – PATIENT RELATIONSHIP

If we are to look at both content and management seriously, it is very difficult to escape the *behavioural implications* for the doctor, the patient, and both the doctor and the patient. If a patient comes in with a sore back and with appropriate offers discusses his marital problems, what is the diagnostic label of this consultation, 'ligamentous sprain', 'marital problem' or both? An unperceptive doctor may have missed the latter, and so in surveying both content and management, we may get false results. Thus if a trial is being done on an analgesic for back pain, the unaware observer may get very poor results by entering inappropriate patients. A failure to gauge the patient's attitudes or personality, or dependency or independency, for example, may lead one to record six consultations for sore throats in the dependent patient, and one in the independent patient.

Studies to observe these characteristics alone are worthwhile, let alone their effects on any conventional research. The effect of different counselling techniques in eliciting problems and meeting patients' needs, is another area which requires careful study. The doctor's own attitudes and prejudices on patient care should be researched, to see the effect on patient care. Do, for example, smoking doctors take poor smoking histories?

THE PROCESS OF THE CONSULTATION

The *process* whereby general practitioners make hypotheses (tentative diagnoses) and test these – *problem solving*, has been one area which has received much attention. Yet one cannot say for certain whether all general practitioners use a common approach. Stop and watch yourself at work. Note how on the basis of your prior knowledge of the patient and the family, epidemiological principles, and the potential seriousness of a disease, for example, you set about dealing with the patient's problems and diseases. Does this vary from patient to patient, or fom symptom to symptom? Meet with a few of your colleagues and interchange ideas, and you may have a paper!

PRACTICE MANAGEMENT

Side room diagnostic tests evolved in practice and used by practitioners should also be evaluated. How useful is the erythrocyte sedimentation rate in the early diagnosis of disease in general practice?

Examination of the management of the practice itself has also been the subject of much attention. Studies on appointment systems, the role of the nurse, off duty arrangements, financial arrangements, suitable facilities, and the like, abound.

All of these have made it much easier for doctors to practise, as have note-taking systems, risks sheets, folders, and so on.

DOCTOR AND PATIENT EDUCATION

If we accept that learning is only of benefit if it is accompanied by a behavioural change, that is, we now change our actions as a result of what we have learned, it is important to analyse those factors which help people change their habits. In a study conducted by our group, it was interesting to learn that patients were not impressed with written data on a subject such as hypertension. Likewise, how much do doctors really learn from didactic lectures, however comfortable they might feel in attending them? How much of their practice behaviour alters as a result of these experiences. All this and other factors have important implications for the training of doctors, and thus for patient care, and as such cannot be neglected.

PRIMARY CARE DELIVERY

In certain areas of the world, there is uncertainty about the role of general practice as a means of delivering primary care. Is general practice the best possible way to meet the patients' and the community's needs? It would appear important, in some communities at least, for general practice to test this hypothesis with an appropriate research model. Implicit in this question is a comparison between general practice and other primary health care systems.

CONCLUSION

In this chapter I have deliberately steered clear from a general review of research in general practice. Instead I have tried to show by means of illustration that there is scope for the active general practitioner to initiate and participate in research. I have done so in the hope of stimulating others, and allaying fears that colleagues may have about the initiation of, or participation in research.

12

The General Family Practice as a Teaching and Learning Environment

WESLEY FABB (AUSTRALIA)

In the previous chapters, attention has been focused on aspects of practice management that directly affect patient care. This chapter examines the potential of the practice, clinic or health centre as a teaching and learning environment for the staff that work there. Even if no special effort is made to focus on teaching and learning, the practice is bound to provide learning experiences. Daily contact with patients and with those who care for them results in learning, often without the individual being very aware of it. However, knowledge of the principles of learning, the provision of simple learning aids, and the organization of the practice to provide additional learning opportunities, can enrich greatly the learning potential of a primary care practice.

PRINCIPLES OF ADULT EDUCATION

The principles of patient education, which have been referred to earlier, and with which many primary care workers are familiar, apply also to staff education. As staff members are adult, certain principles of adult education apply: (Fabb, Heffernan, Phillips and Stone, 1976).

1. Adults value the opportunity to evaluate their performance against a standard
Most people are concerned about how they measure up. This applies just as much to administrative staff as it does to the health care professionals. Thus members of the clinic staff should be given the opportunity to have their performance evaluated. This can be done by observing their work, by a written assessment using prepared forms, or by using self-assessment techniques. Immediate feedback by the assessor and discussion will identify strengths and weaknesses. Specified weaknesses may become the focus for subsequent learning exercises. Most professionals are dissatisfied with their deficiencies, if they believe they are relevant to their daily work, and are motivated to remedy them.

Although the concept of staff assessment is a simple one, and its implementation straightforward, how often is it carried out in the practice, clinic or health centre? How often is the performance of the receptionist, secretary, practice nurse, social worker or doctor evaluated? However it is done, it should be as non-threatening as possible. The purpose of evaluation is to critique, not to criticize. If helpful critiques are given, the process will be accepted and enjoyed.

2. *Having identified deficiencies, adults prefer to select their own learning experiences and methods.*

Most adults prefer to be self-directing. Of course, many graduates of academic institutions emerge as educational cripples having been subject to an authoritarian, directive, and at times oppressive educational environment. Like the dependent patient, they need to be gently weaned from their dependency and encouraged to take responsibility for their own learning. Once they have become accustomed to the joys of self-directed learning, they will establish this as a lifelong habit.

It is unfortunate that the concept of self-directed learning has been misunderstood by many people. It is not leaving the learner without advice, guidance or assistance. Knowles, the most prominent proponent of self-directed learning puts it very well when he says: (Knowles, 1975a)

> *'In its broadest meaning "self-directed learning" describes a process in which individuals take the initiative, with or without the help of others, in diagnosing their learning needs, formulating learning goals, identifying human and material resources for learning, choosing and implementing appropriate learning strategies, and evaluating learning outcomes. Other labels found in the literature to describe this process are "self-planned learning", "inquiry method", "independent learning", "self-education", "self-instruction", "self-teaching", "self-study", and "autonomous learning". The trouble with most of these labels is that they seem to imply learning in isolation, whereas self-directed learning usually takes place in association with various kinds of helpers, such as teachers, tutors, mentors, resource people and peers. There is a lot of mutuality among a group of self-directed learners.'*

Self-directed learning gives the learner the opportunity to develop his own learning style and to learn in the way which best suits his personality and his process of thinking.

The clinic which is committed to the continuing education of its staff will provide the facilities, opportunities and resources, both human and material, to enable its staff to pursue their own learning direction. Ways in which this can be done will be detailed later.

3. *Adults prefer a problem oriented approach to learning*

Learning experiences which seem remote from the demands of the job will have little attraction for adults. Schoolchildren suffer this sort of experience much of the time, but adults need to see the *relevance* to their daily work of what they are learning. Moreover, learning takes place more readily if based upon actual problems which occur on the job.

The receptionist will be interested in the question: 'How do you determine priorities of urgency when dealing with telephone calls requesting medical care?' The social worker will respond to the question: 'What are the facilities in this community for the treatment of alcoholism?', and the doctor to the question: 'What are the indications for using a beta-blocker in hypertension?'

Problems which entail a description of an actual situation almost invariably attract interest. For example, the following problem would be of interest to medical staff: 'A 32-year old man suffering from chest pain which, on the history, is not cardiac, is very anxious about his condition as his father died of a heart attack at the age of 42. What steps should be taken to exclude cardiac disease and counsel the patient?' The administrative staff would be interested in the problem of the middle-aged woman who repeatedly brings her children to the clinic without notice, always at the end of the surgery, and who complains if she has to wait. Almost always the children have trivial complaints, but on one occasion her eldest child did have a serious illness for which treatment was delayed because the receptionist had refused an appointment. Such problems can be drawn from the rich daily experiences of the community based primary care unit.

4. *Adults respond best when the learning situation is not threatening and where there is a good relationship between the teacher and the learner*

Anxiety in small doses is a good stimulus to learning, but in excess it can be disabling and severely inhibit learning. If the clinic or practice is to be a congenial learning environment, all involved should strive to be helpful, considerate and kind to each other. A sharp rebuke for a mistake may sometimes be necessary, but in general, a gentle approach gets much better results. If a staff member is afraid and threatened by his or her superiors, it may be almost impossible to share problems and queries, so that mistakes will continue and little learning will occur. Senior members of staff should remember the awe in which many juniors hold them and recognize that this may inhibit communication.

If the clinic staff consciously and purposefully set about to create open, honest communication between staff members, and develop an atmosphere of trust, the potential of the environment for learning will increase immeasurably. Knowles places great emphasis on the importance of *climate setting* prior to learning (Knowles, 1975b). This applies not only to specific educational events, but to the daily work atmosphere as well.

5. *Adults like to know regularly how they are progressing*

It has already been noted that adults like to have opportunities for evaluating their performance. This is not a static process. Regular progress assessment with timely and constructive feedback is needed and valued. This especially applies to the new member of the clinic, no matter at what level he or she is working. Assessment should not be confined to the technical aspects of staff members' work, but should also apply to the quality of their interpersonal relationships with others in the practice, with colleagues outside of the practice, and with the patients. The importance of the interpersonal dimension cannot be overemphasized, as it is in this area that so many problems arise.

Regular progress assessment will not occur unless the clinic staff agree that it should, and unless one or more people are specifically designated to be responsible for ensuring that it takes place.

6. *Adults want to immediately apply newly acquired knowledge and skills*
Adults find little attraction in learning for the remote future. They prefer to be able to use tomorrow what they learn today. Discussions and other educational events should therefore focus on the here and now problems relevant to the everyday work of the staff.

Of course we all have to learn about less common events or conditions, some of which we may not encounter for some time. Perhaps the best time to discuss such topics is immediately after they have occurred in the practice or in the district. How to cope with an outbreak of scabies will be learned much faster after the first couple of cases have mystified the practice staff. Likewise, knowledge about meningococcal meningitis will be much more readily learned after the first reported case at the nearby Army barracks.

7. *Adults like helping others to learn*
There is the 'teacher' in most of us. It is not necessary to call in droves of expert resource personnel to teach the clinic staff. Each person has a special set of skills and knowledge, and most people are only too happy to pass these on. Even if a staff member is not a 'full bottle' on a subject, he or she soon will be if given the time, resources and encouragement to study the subject with a view to presenting it to other staff members. Most excellent presentations may result from this type of approach. Moreover, the act of preparing such a presentation is a very potent learning experience in itself.

A less formal way of sharing knowledge is in group discussion – a method which has been repeatedly demonstrated to be an effective learning process. However, it works optimally only if all participants are given the opportunity to contribute and if their contribution is respected by the others in the group. In a practice where there are more than four members, regular group discussions can be amongst the most useful learning exercises which can be carried out. Group discussions work best when all participants regard themselves as learners, even the teacher or the resource person.

Group discussions have an important part to play in attitude change. Often an individual's attitude will be changed during group discussion, although rigidly held for a long time previously.

HOW CAN THE PRACTICE PROVIDE EDUCATIONAL OPPORTUNITIES

There are many ways, some very simple and inexpensive, of providing educational opportunities. Some occur in most practices informally and almost without being noticed. Some of these methods will be detailed below, with examples of their use.

Introduction and orientation activities

These are really educational activities. They have been mentioned in earlier chapters on the health team and on health records.

Whenever a new staff member arrives, or whenever a new system or facility is introduced into a practice, a means of introducing and orienting the member, or introducing the facility, should be devised. Personal introduction and oral explanation of the job to the newcomer is commonplace. A very effective adjunct to this is to present the new staff member with a manual describing in detail the philosophy, policy and procedures of the practice, the services offered, and the staff and facilities provided. Many practices now have such a manual and its use in the orientation of new staff has been very successful, so much so that all practices, clinics and health centres would be well advised to prepare and use regularly such a manual.

In addition, a detailed, specific and unambiguous description of the tasks to be carried out by the newcomer is a vital ingredient to the successful integration and effective performance of the individual. How often is a new staff member criticized for defaulting on a task without ever knowing that this was his or her task in the first place?

Sometimes very simple and obvious information may be vital to the newcomer. For example, billing patients after hours may be very threatening to the new young doctor until he is told what procedure to use. Using prescription forms for the first time may be very frightening for the doctor who has only ever worked in a hospital. Knowing how to get help after hours and to whom to refer difficult cases is important information to the novitiate, although commonplace to the established doctors in the practice. Attention to this sort of detail will avoid many difficulties and much anxiety.

In introducing new staff, it is important to allow enough time to assimilate all the new information presented to them. In the same way as we often expect patients to remember lengthy instructions (and so often they don't), we also seem to expect the new staff member to learn it all at one sitting. Several weeks, even months, may be needed for the adjustment process. This applies not just to the process of learning the job, but also to the process of relating to others in the clinic. To ask regularly how the newcomer is fitting in, and particularly how he or she is *feeling* about the job, the other staff and the practice, will always be worthwhile. Often hidden fears and anxieties surface in this process, most of which can be easily resolved. The essential elements are sufficient time and a friendly and open approach so that the individual feels comfortable about airing any problems, no matter how seemingly trivial or 'foolish'. To attempt this process in a brisk, hurried and impatient way is a waste of time, and indeed is worse than doing nothing at all. In essence, what is being suggested is that the best features of a good doctor–patient relationship should be transferred to this situation.

On-the-spot consultations

These are commonplace in clinical practice. They occur between medical staff, other health professionals and administrative staff. The value of such encounters could be enhanced by giving attention to the process of the interchange. Several questioning styles have been described, each of which can be used to fit the occasion, (RCGP, 1972). The first is called the *authoritarian* style which consists of giving a direct answer to a question. This is often inappropriate, but sometimes is essential. In an emergency, a question asking the correct dose of a drug to be given urgently deserves a direct and immediate response. In less urgent situations, and when time pressures are not great, other approaches may be much more appropriate. The *Socratic* approach involves the well-known question and answer technique – the teacher questions and the learner answers. By carefully framing and sequencing questions, the learner is led towards the answer and the solution.

The so-called '*heuristic*' approach is one where the questioner and the questioned explore the problem together, each contributing to the building up of an answer to the question or a solution to the problem.

Finally, the *counselling* approach may be the most appropriate style of questioning when it seems as if there is a considerable emotional element in the problem. Maybe the difficulty is largely the emotional response of the health worker. By exploring this with a counselling approach which examines feelings as well as thoughts, the learner can become aware of the emotional side of the interaction with the patient and thus cope with the problem more effectively.

So those casual, informal, almost unnoticed consultations between health workers in the corridor or over morning tea can become much more meaningful and helpful and yet still remain pleasantly informal if the above-mentioned techniques are used. Those interested in exploring this subject further would benefit from reading the relevant section in *The Future General Practitioner* (RCGP, 1972)

Observation of the staff member's work

This evaluative process can occur at any level in the practice. Doctors can observe each other; a trainee doctor or medical student can observe his supervisor or vice versa; nurses, social workers or other health professionals can observe each other at work, and the administrative staff can do likewise.

We all know how helpful it is to have someone looking over our shoulder when we are learning something new, provided the observer's approach is helpful and facilitates our learning. The observer has to resist the temptation to interfere or take over (unless of course the patient is at risk). The observer should remember his or her early fumbling efforts and how quickly expertise was acquired through practice.

Trainee doctors and medical students have found it helpful to observe experienced doctors at work, and with special training they can gain deep insight into the process of the consultation.

On the other hand, the value of an experienced clinician observing a trainee or medical student is well documented from many countries. In North America this commonplace event is carried out through one-way mirrors or by video camera to a remote TV monitor. The observer uses a rating form, an abundance of which exist. Rating forms can be fashioned to observe and measure any aspect of the consultation process. Slavish use of standard forms may result in some aspects of the consultation being overlooked or under-rated. For example, on one occasion a trainee may desire the attention of the observer to be focused on his questioning style, on another occasion on his non-verbal signals, and on yet another occasion on the quality of his communication in explaining, advising and counselling the patient.

When a video recording can be made, the individual being observed has the advantage of being able to see himself as others see him. This can be a salutory experience as one witnesses the unintended non-verbal signals, the odd mannerisms, or the patient's comments that went unheard or unacknowledged. An extension of this process devised by Kagan (Kagan, 1975) involves replay of the video recording in the company of a person trained to assist the subject to identify the thoughts and feelings which existed during the interview. This process, called interpersonal process recall, has been most helpful to those learning consulting and counselling skills. It enables the individual to recognize, acknowledge and accept the inter-relatedness of intellectual and emotional factors in the patient, the health care professional, and in their relationship. This knowledge can be used in refining consulting and counselling skills to the advantage of both the health care professional and the patient.

The process of observation can be applied equally well to the procedural area as it can to the consultation. Often a helpful, encouraging or reassuring word can boost confidence as the learner struggles to make his or her fingers do what looks so easy when the expert does it. Sometimes a demonstration is the best way of proceeding, followed by the novice repeating what the teacher has done. This method is so commonplace that no more needs to be said about it.

The valuable process of observation should not be confined to the health care professionals. It can be very effective if used with other staff. The novice receptionist would benefit greatly from having an experienced receptionist observe her work and then discuss it with her. The most important element in the process is the discussion afterwards, and again the atmosphere in which this occurs is of critical importance. Unless the climate is friendly, warm and facilitating, the exercise will be largely a waste of time.

It should be mentioned in passing that filling the 'teacher' role is probably one of the most effective ways of learning and contributes substantially to the continuing education of the teacher.

Case discussion

The discussion of clinical cases with a colleague is a commonplace event. Benefit would be derived by introducing an element of structure into such discussions. How often are such discussions desultory and diffuse? The simple process of beginning by stating clearly the objective of the discussion would enhance both the effectiveness and the efficiency of the discourse which followed. To begin by saying 'I need advice on how to change a patient from an oral hypoglycaemic onto insulin', would orient the discussion from the outset. The clinical features would then be described, questions asked and answered, the problem clearly defined in all its dimensions, and then solved expeditiously. If neither party has the full information needed, other colleagues or references can be consulted.

A similar process can occur in a group where several health workers discuss a problem. The suggested procedure of setting objectives still applies. The value of several opinions often exceeds that of one.

Sometimes the boot is on the other foot. The supervisor may initiate the discussion to see how the trainee or learner is progressing or how he or she is coping with selected problems. A 'difficult patient' of the practice may be selected to test the understanding of the learner. The process described above still applies. The supervisor can state the objectives at the outset so that both know what is expected.

The importance of objective setting in educational activities cannot be overemphasized. When all agree on what the objectives are and the task is, progress is facilitated.

Medical record review

This process is similar in many ways to case discussion, but there are some important differences, the most obvious of which is the inspection of the record itself. This can give insight into the individual's problem solving process, knowledge of the condition, and skill and diligence in record keeping. If records are poor, one can only conclude that the recorder has done a poor job of recording. One cannot assume his or her other clinical processes are equally poor, although in the chapter on health records it is suggested that there is a positive relationship between the quality of the record and the quality of patient care provided.

Given that the records are well kept, they can be used as a basis for discussing the problem solving approach adopted, the conclusions reached, the level of certainty of those conclusions, the actions taken or planned, the education, advice and instructions given to the patient, the proposed follow-up, and the individual's knowledge of the patient's problem or condition in physical, psychological and social terms. Cases can be selected for discussion randomly or according to a prepared plan. Stephen Smith's tracer technique (Smith, 1977), which focuses on the management of specific conditions such as hypertension or diabetes, also can be used.

Using a medical record as the basis for discussion makes it easy to ask such questions as, 'What do you expect the chest X-ray to show you?' or 'Why did you order a complete biochemical profile?' or 'If this test result is abnormal, what will you do; in what way will it alter your management of this patient and in what way will it alter your thinking or feeling about the problem?'

The use of a well-kept record system is strongly advocated and the use of the problem-oriented approach has been shown to be very helpful to many clinicians. It is not universally accepted, but those who have used it successfully would not revert to their old style. As pointed out in the chapter on health records, it is not the problem-oriented medical record system that makes good records; it helps, but the essential ingredient is the problem-oriented disciplined mental apparatus of the user.

Needless to say, in a large practice, clinic or health centre, records would be used by health workers other than doctors and could be used for discussion in the same way, either on an individual basis or in a group.

Audiotaping of consultations

This educational method is coming into vogue as a simple, inexpensive way of gaining insight into one's consulting process. Having obtained the permission of the patient (preferably recording this on the tape), the tape recorder is allowed to run during the entire consultation. Extensive experience in the United Kingdom has shown that in most instances it is soon forgotten by both the patient and the health care professional, and does not intrude on their interaction. It can be left on for a whole consulting session if desired, after which it can be reviewed either by the individual health care professional or by a group. In many ways this is a more accurate way of reviewing what happened in the consultation than examining the medical record.

The method of analysis of these recordings has been well described by Byrne and Long (Byrne and Long, 1976). Much benefit can be derived by noting the style of questioning of the doctor, the responses of the patient, and the use of such techniques as silence, encouraging noises, confrontation, and so on. It is salutary to hear one's poorly framed and sequenced questions, the unheard or unacknowledged patient response or question, or the inadequate explanation given. This process can lead to more effective ways of conducting the consultation and is strongly recommended to all trainees, and even to experienced doctors.

An extension of this method is to type up a transcript of the interview, which is sometimes even more revealing of inadequacies in the consulting process.

Such recordings or transcripts can be examined by the individual or discussed with a colleague or in a group. The latter is rather more threatening and thus a suitable climate must be created in the group which encourages and applauds open, honest communication and a fair critique of the individual's performance. It is a critique, not criticism which is needed, accompanied by helpful advice and support which will enable the individual to perform better in the future. Such groups would be akin to Balint groups and a similar group atmosphere is needed.

This method is one of the most promising to arise in recent years and it is hoped that it will become a regular exercise for all health care professionals.

Practice tutorials

The ideal of holding regular practice tutorials may seem a little *avant-garde* to some, but this is already happening in many places all around the world. Regular tutorials are held, often at lunch time, and attended by medical and allied health professionals, and sometimes by other staff as well. Often a resource person is selected from the practice staff, and occasionally from outside. The topic is usually chosen by the group.

This sort of activity is to' be strongly encouraged as it provides yet another opportunity for staff members to obtain their continuing education in the practice environment. There is merit in this type of activity being developed for the administrative staff as well.

To ensure the success of practice tutorials, a diligent, efficient coordinator is needed to take responsibility for organizing the activity. The staff should be involved in the selection of topics relevant to their daily work, staff members should be used as resource persons whenever appropriate, and the group discussion format should be encouraged as much as possible. A short presentation which focuses on actual patients' problems, followed by questions and discussion, is ideal. A useful collection of case histories for discussion is now available in book form (Fabb and Marshall, 1983)

The value and interest of the presentation is enhanced by using visual aids, either in the form of 35mm transparencies or overhead projector transparencies, and of course the old black or white board still has its place. Schematic drawings, flow charts and easy-to-remember lists all aid memory retention. The occasional movie film or video recording can be most valuable, provided it is well produced and does not present just a 'talking head'. Moving pictures are essential when movement has to be demonstrated, such as in the carrying out of physical examination or procedures, or in depicting a clinical consultation. The use of graphics in such presentations enhances their value, provided the graphics are congruent and synchronous with the spoken word. It is distracting and confusing to have the written word out-of-kilter with the spoken word. Moreover, the written graphics should be very simple, short and crystal clear.

Practice clinical meetings

These are a little different from tutorials. Cases involving patients of the practice are discussed in order to design improved management schedules for individual patients. Although they can be time-consuming, if objectives are set, unnecessary and irrelevant discussion curtailed, solutions and action plans developed, and tasks assigned, they can be invaluable. Follow-up discussion at later meetings will reveal the wisdom of the decisions reached and any corrective action needed.

The meetings serve another useful purpose. They facilitate the communication process between health workers. The communication network becomes extremely complex with a large number of health workers, and specific efforts need to be made to overcome the difficulties inherent therein.

The meetings are educational for all concerned and are highly relevant to individual patient care, usually in the widest possible context of the community as well as in the narrower clinical context.

Practice administrative meetings

Although these may be viewed as primarily administrative, it is hard to separate administrative functions from patient care. These meetings occur in many practices and should be encouraged. In some practices the whole staff proceed to a restaurant for lunch every month or two, leaving only a reliever to man the switchboard. In this more congenial and relaxed environment, aided by a bottle or two of wine, many practice problems can be sorted out. The social setting appears to break down interpersonal barriers which may exist in the practice.

Although there is ample justification for the principals or owners of the practice meeting separately to discuss financial, administrative and staff matters, the involvement of administrative staff in meetings as described above builds up goodwill, engenders cooperation, and often results in the advent of very good ideas, sometimes from the most unexpected source.

Visits to outside practices or health facilities

The educational opportunities for practice staff members need not be confined to the precincts of the practice. Visits to nearby practices and dialogue with those working there can be of great value. Ideas can be exchanged, different ways of doing things observed, and common problems shared. It is often comforting to know that someone else doing the same job has similar difficulties, problems and frustrations. All categories of staff member would benefit from such visits. Reciprocating the situation by having staff from another practice visit one's own practice can also be mutually beneficial.

Visits should not be confined, however, to other practices. Visits to other health facilities such as infant welfare centres, geriatric centres, rehabilitation units, hospitals and other health agencies can not only enhance understanding of what these agencies do, but also can establish a personal relationship between practice staff and the staff of the agencies visited. This often breaks down the barriers created by ignorance and prejudice and results in a more effective use of these agencies for the benefit of the patient and a more cooperative attitude between the staff in both situations.

Still another group of organizations well worth visiting are industrial, commercial and municipal installations. In some areas, industrial or occupational health is very important. A visit to local factories or manufacturing concerns gives insight into the working conditions that exist there, the safety measures employed, the potential for improving safety and protecting workers from injuries such as back strain or eye injury, and the role and function of the industrial nurse or doctor where they are employed. Again, better understanding and better relationships are engendered.

Visits to food manufacturing establishments will reveal what stringent measures are taken to avoid contamination. Health workers can see for themselves the physical proximity of workers to the food being processed and can therefore more readily advise workers with infections about the need for time off or temporary removal from food processing.

Visits to municipal installations such as water purification and sewage disposal units give insight into how the community is provided with these basic amenities which have done so much to improve health, yet are often forgotten.

During such visits as described above, the focus would appropriately be on the prevention of accidents or illness and hopefully may result in improvement in safety measures.

Another aspect of such visits could be discussion with administrative staff about the processing of worker's compensation claims and sick leave certificates. Better understanding of mutual problems can result in improved administrative procedures.

The practice library or resource centre

If a practice, clinic or health centre is to realize fully its potential as an educational environment, a library or resource centre is essential. The term 'resource centre' is to be preferred, as in addition to books and periodicals, audiovisual resources such as audiotapes, 35mm slides, charts, illustrations, flow charts and even films and videotapes should be included, together with the equipment needed to use these resources. This will be mentioned later.

A quiet area is to be preferred. Furnishing the staff tea room with library shelves and equipment is a poor substitute for a separate room where any staff member can work without being disturbed. Someone should be appointed to take responsibility for the library resources and equipment, and to order material required for use in practice educational activities or for individual use. A small catalogue is needed, and an honour system for borrowing usually works well in this confined environment. Spare globes for projection equipment and a service arrangement for repairs are essential to the smooth functioning of a resource centre.

An extension of this concept is the provision of reading and viewing facilities for patient education. The provision of pamphlets and booklets has been mentioned in the chapter on patient education. Some practices are now providing tape/slide or video programmes on health matters in waiting rooms or in separate carrell type facilities. This can save the health worker a lot of time in explanation, and programmes can be repeated as often as the patient wishes.

Research activities

Although research may not be seen as an educational activity, it clearly is. There is a pressing need to further research the discipline of family medicine. Research can be epidemiological, clinical or operational. There are innumerable studies which need to be carried out.

Epidemiological research is important as it provides the practice and the individual health worker with a profile of the variety of problems and conditions which present. This is a useful starting point for the development of educational programmes. The practice profile will indicate the topics suitable for practice tutorials, the individual profile will indicate the areas on which the individual should concentrate in devising his or her own educational programme. By noting those problems or conditions with which the individual is having difficulty, learning objectives can be formulated and a remedial programme developed.

Epidemiological research can also unearth hitherto unexpected associations as Robin Pinsent has shown in his studies. The community based practice is very advantageously placed to observe the interaction between man and his environment – *human ecology*. However, accurate and systematic observation and recording is necessary. This can be done with manual systems, the E book being a classical example, but the advent of the in-house computer will assist this immeasurably as is indicated in Chapter 10. Its capacity to manipulate data in a few microseconds constitutes an enormous advantage over manual systems.

Clinical research can be divided broadly into two categories. The first is the natural history of illness and its response to therapy. There is no need to elaborate on the rich variety of opportunities available for this type of research. There is so much more that we need to know about health and disease in all its physical, psychological and social dimensions, that no one wanting to carry out this sort of research should find any difficulty in selecting a suitable area for study.

The second category is what can be usefully described as '*process research*'. It focuses on *how* health care professionals carry out their professional tasks. There is a great need for research into the processes of the consultation, problem solving and decision making, counselling, family therapy, group therapy and so on. How do we solve clinical problems and make clinical decisions? Is there an optimal way of conducting a consultation, and if so, what is it? These questions are but partly answered. This area appears to be one of the most fruitful for research in clinical practice at the present time and such research should be encouraged. It would also be an educational exercise of the greatest possible benefit to the researcher as well as to his reading audience.

'*Operational research*' is a term used here to indicate that area of research which studies the systems the practice uses. This sort of research can provide answers to such questions as: 'Is the appointment system or the accounting system or the stock control system optimally efficient?' Research into the way in which health services are provided, both in the microcosm of the practice, clinic or health centre, and in the macrocosm of the community, is of great contemporary importance in many countries. How many systems of health care delivery are operating at maximum efficiency? Study of these systems can lead to improvements. This area of research can be of particular interest to administrative staff.

To conclude, it is worth reiterating that research is an educational experience and can enrich greatly the practice as a learning environment. But it needs someone in the practice to initiate and coordinate research, obtaining where necessary the advice and resources needed.

Evaluative activity

Evaluation is part of education. Before learning begins, it is useful to evaluate what is already known so that strengths and weaknesses can be identified. After learning, evaluation is again important to determine progress and identify further areas of deficiency.

Evaluation has been mentioned earlier in the section on the principles of adult learning. All professionals worth their salt desire evaluation, and thus it should be an integral part of practice activities. In those practices which are also teaching units, evaluation is a prominent feature. Some methods of evaluation such as observation and audio and videotaping have already been mentioned.

In some teaching units, formal evaluation is carried out annually. The methods employed are based on those used by colleges and academies of general practitioners and family physicians. A good example is the Annual In-Service Examination conducted in the Department of Family Practice at the Medical University of South Carolina by John Corley (Corley, 1976). Multi-choice questions, written simulations such as patient management problems, simulated interviews, physical examinations and variants of these tests are used. The concept is catching on in North America and it seems likely to become a feature of many family practice training programmes. A text on assessing clinical competence by Fabb and Marshall (1983) is a useful reference.

However, there is another aspect of evaluation which is less prominent, although not less important. It addresses itself to such questions as: 'What are the expectations of patients visiting this practice and to what extent are they being met?', 'What are the expectations of staff members in this practice and to what extent are they being met?', 'What is the most important expectation of each group and how can we measure the extent to which it has been achieved?', and 'What are the most important indicators of the viability and growth of the practice and how can they be maximized?' Answers to these questions help the practice to perceive the need for changes to its policies, operating procedures and personnel behaviour. A set of methodological procedures for such evaluations has been developed (Heffernan, 1978a,b).

The importance of this type of evaluation cannot be stressed too strongly. How many patients are dissatisfied with the services they receive? Do we know why? To what extent do staff members feel fulfilled and satisfied with their role? To answer these questions is a pressing requirement for the 1980s and beyond. Again, this activity is educational in essence and can lead only to the enrichment of the practice staff affected by such activity.

Access to outside educational activity

In most countries, there is a superabundance of educational activity in the health care field. Perhaps more than in most other professions, continuing education is seen as an important part of the professional life of health care workers. Whereas much of this is provided out of practice hours at nights and weekends, there is an increasing and laudable tendency to hold such events during working hours. Half-day release programmes for trainees and an educational half-day for practising professionals are becoming more commonplace. Such programmes identify education as part of the working week. Practices, clinics and health centres are becoming increasingly aware of the advantage of allowing, indeed encouraging, staff to attend such events. Although they have been available for medical staff for eons, it is only in recent times that educational events and courses have been available for receptionists, medical secretaries and other office staff. These have been enthusiastically accepted and well attended. Their further development should be encouraged.

Little more needs to be said about educational activity outside the practice except to underscore the need to encourage staff attendance and to make it easy for staff to do so. The maintenance of the salary of the staff member during such attendance, and even the payment of course fees by the practice, will demonstrate the commitment of the practice to continuing education for **all** its staff.

The computer and education

For years we have talked about the imminent appearance of the computer in medical practice. Now it is here. With the advent of the microprocessor, it is predicted that computers will be installed in most practices, especially the larger clinics and health centres, within the next ten years. The technicalities of this subject have been dealt with in Chapter 10 and so the remarks here will be confined to the educational uses of the computer.

To begin with, the computer can be used like a reference book. Data such as, for example, drug data can be recorded and recalled at the command of the health worker in a few seconds. This will be much easier and faster than thumbing through a book and therefore will be much more likely to be used. The less one has to do to get information, the more often it will be sought and used.

A similar function is the recording and recall of the patient's history on computer. This has been mentioned in Chapters 8 and 10. A more sophisticated function is the manipulation of this information to give data on morbidity, treatment schedules, the results of treatment, and similar data. This type of information is educational as it assists the user to learn the morbidity patterns, the outcomes of treatment, and his prescribing patterns, which he can then compare with those of others in the practice.

A more sophisticated use of the computer is as an aid in diagnosis. Protocols for questioning or flow charts for problem solving and decision making can be entered into the computer and easily recalled to assist the clinician to ask the appropriate questions in the optimal sequence. In this process, the computer does not manipulate the data elicited – it simply provides a guide for the clinician to improve his diagnostic and therapeutic efficiency and effectiveness. There are already in existence manual systems which, however, are not as convenient or fast to use as the computer system.

An even more sophisticated use of the computer is its use in processing patient data to arrive at the diagnostic probabilities. This is a very complex application, is only partly developed to date, and is likely to be of maximum use in physical diagnosis. Where it has been used for this purpose (de Dombal, Leaper, Horrocks, Staniland and McCann 1974), it has markedly improved the accuracy of diagnosis. Its application in psychological medicine is still a long way off. The difficulty of entering soft data such as non-verbal signals seems to preclude early developments in this area. It seems that the most feasible contemporary use of the computer in diagnosis will be in displaying short subroutines for diagnosis and management, particularly in the physical area.

Turning now to the more obviously educational applications of the computer, it can be used to store multi-choice questions and programmed patient management problems for the use of the clinical staff. The

multi-choice questions could be accompanied by correct answers, explana-
tory notes and references, and could be supplied on tapes or flexible discs
for use and return to a resource centre. Academic bodies could produce
such tapes or discs regularly to update the clinician with the latest
advances.

Programmed patient management problems require a computer which
has the memory capacity to cope with complex branching problems. In
these problems, the user is given a brief description of a clinical situation
and then asked to select from a number of management options such as
taking a history, conducting a physical examination, or carrying out
investigations. Having made a choice, the user is instructed to proceed to
the relevant clinical section, where he can elicit data from hundreds of
items of history, or physical examination, or investigations. As he asks for
each item of information, which he does by entering a specific code into the
computer terminal, the answer is displayed by the computer either on a
visual display unit or in printed form. With each new piece of information,
the user makes decisions about what further information he requires, thus
proceeding through the problem as in clinical practice until a diagnostic
conclusion is reached and treatment implemented. Because the user
interacts with the computer, a variety of pathways for the user to take must
be provided. For example, in an emergency problem, the treatment
provided by the user determines the patient's response. Thus allowance
has to be made for inappropriate as well as appropriate treatment. In the
former case, the user would be told that the patient had deteriorated and
would be directed to another part of the problem where there may be an
opportunity to retrieve the situation. These patient management problems
are of great educational value as they mimic the real clinical situation so
closely. They can be used by individuals or by a group. Group discussion
of these problems has been shown to be a very fruitful educational
experience.

When the problem is completed, the computer can print out the
pathway taken by the user, the clinical data elicited and in what sequence,
the outcome of any treatment given, and a comparison between the user's
performance and that of the optimal management as determined by a
criterion group. The user's performance can be given a numeric score to
give him some idea of how he compares with the criterion group. In
addition, the problem can be accompanied by a commentary on the actual
case and its management and outcome, as well as an account of the most
efficient and effective diagnostic approach to the presenting symptoms or
signs, and the accepted contemporary treatment routine.

Great potential exists for the future development of this concept and
academic institutions should be planning to produce this material. A very
recent development is the recording 'chip' which records the user's steps
and which can be sent to the academic institution for assessment and
comment as part of the process of periodic review of professional standards.

PROFESSIONAL STANDARDS REVIEW IN A PRACTICE SETTING

Woven throughout the preceding pages are descriptions of a number of ways of reviewing professional standards. Observation of staff members, case discussion, medical record review, group discussions, research, evaluation, and computerized tests are some of the methods which can be used. In this section, the concept of professional standards review, with special emphasis on its application in a practice setting, will be further expanded.

A number of terms have come into popular use, in describing professional standards review, but the meaning they carry seems to vary. For the purpose of clarity, brief definitions will be given here. Peer review is a general term used to describe the process of assessment by which peers continuously judge each other (ACHS, AMA and AHA, 1978). Clinical review is that part of the process of peer review related to clinical practice. Clinical review is subdivided into two parts: The first part is quality assurance which implies assessment of medical practice and administration to provide information about the quality and appropriateness of care, and a commitment to corrective action where care does not meet the criteria of quality; in other words to assure quality of care. The second part

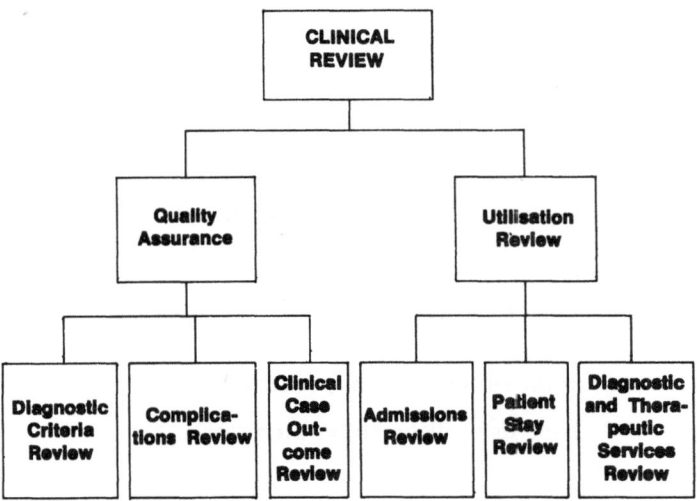

Figure 1   The elements of formal systems of clinical review. Reproduced with the permission of the Australian Council on Hospital Standards, the Australian Medical Association, and the Australian Hospital Association

is utilization review which comprises the measurement of the use of institutional resources in order to ensure that care is delivered in the most economical way consistent with quality, and that available resources are allocated in the most efficient way.

Quality assurance is further subdivided into diagnostic criteria review, complications review and clinical case outcome review. Utilization review is subdivided into admissions review, patient stay review and diagnostic and therapeutic services review (see Figure 1). Although the first two are strictly institutional measures which may be applicable to medical staff who admit patients to hospital, the latter – diagnostic and therapeutic services review – is applicable to the practice, clinic or health centre, as well as to the hospital. A review of the use of diagnostic and therapeutic facilities in the practice will reveal whether they are being under or over utilized, whether they are being used economically and efficiently, how cost-effective they are, what financial benefits accrue to the practice from their use, and whether the employment of skilled technical staff to use the facilities is justified on economic grounds. Whilst this is an educational exercise which could indicate a need for behavioural change in members of the practice staff, it is principally of administrative significance and will not be further detailed here.

Returning to the concept of clinical review, attention will now be given to *criteria auditing*, which is a method of conducting formal review. It requires the establishment of criteria which are objective definitions of each aspect of the quality of care, in order to determine whether these criteria of care are being met. *Medical record review* is a common method used to do this, but direct observation, case review and discussion could serve the same purpose.

The process of criteria audit comprises several steps:

1. Choose a topic for review.
2. Develop criteria in respect of the topic.
3. Assess what occurs in practice.
4. Evaluate whether the criteria are being met.
5. Take corrective action if they are not being met.
6. Reassess later to determine if the corrective action has resulted in the required improvement.
7. Repeat steps 5 and 6 until the required standards are reached.

How can criteria audit be applied in practice?

Each step in the above list will be elaborated upon.

Choosing the topic for review

The choice of topic will best be left to the practice staff, either individually or collectively. To ensure success in criteria audit, steps should be taken to ensure that all staff members agree to the topic. Otherwise resistance may prevent a satisfactory outcome. Typical topics could include the diagnosis, investigation and management of urinary tract infections, sore throat, hypertension, anxiety or depression. Topics may focus on individual diseases, procedures, investigations, incidents (such as delayed messages) or the complications of treatment in a particular unit, such as for example, wound infections in the practice theatre.

In selecting topics it is wise to avoid controversial subjects or uncommonly occurring conditions. Also the number of cases to be reviewed should be decided, and over what period, in order to assess the subject adequately.

In hospitals, clinical review committees will carry out some of these tasks; there may be merit in selecting a similar small group in the practice to do the same. Certainly at least one person would need to be given this specific responsibility.

Developing criteria in respect of the topic

The criteria should also be developed by the practice staff. There may be some who would protest that this will result in low standards, as people would tend to set not too difficult a target to reach. Experience suggests that this is not so and that high standards will be set. An interesting study in Canada has been carried out in which individual practitioners set their own standards for criteria review (Clark and Putnam, 1977).

It is the responsibility of academic organizations to assist in this process by drawing up criteria which they consider appropriate to guide practitioners in their selection which, however, must be modified to suit the location of the practice and the services and facilities available.

In developing criteria, one should use clear, specific definitions so that the presence or absence of the criteria can be easily identified; limit the number to twenty or less to keep the process manageable; and communicate the criteria to all relevant staff, allowing time for amendments, so that all agree on the criteria before they are applied.

The form in which criteria are described is becoming standardized for hospital audits. A similar format could apply to practice audit. The first part of the standard form focuses on the *justification for the diagnosis and management of the condition including surgery or special diagnostic or therapeutic procedures* and, where appropriate, the *justification for admission to hospital*, in other words the *process* of care. The second part focuses on the *outcome of treatment including the mortality, the duration of treatment, and the complications*. If the patient is admitted to hospital, the period in hospital and the discharge status are included. The *standard* is set at 0% or 100%. Thus no cases should meet certain criteria and all cases should meet the other criteria. For example, in the correct management of iron deficiency anaemia, there should be a 0% mortality and a 100% satisfactory response. With respect to some criteria, exceptions are specified.

Using the iron deficiency example again, packed red cell transfusion should be used in 0% of cases *except* if the haemoglobin is below 5g% or if congestive cardiac failure is present. Wherever an exception is listed, a definition of the exception (and instructions for data retrieval when record review is the vehicle for audit), is given. The exception of congestive cardiac failure mentioned above is defined as clinical or X-ray evidence of peripheral or pulmonary oedema, basal rales, ventricular gallop and a third heart sound. Figure 2 illustrates a typical set of audit criteria for iron deficiency anaemia.

Although this figure relates to the hospital care of iron deficiency anaemia, it could easily be modified to suit a community based practice. Much work needs to be done in developing audit criteria for the wide range of conditions seen in general family practice. The technique of 'criteria mapping' seems particularly promising (Greenfield, Kaplan, Goldberg, Nadler and Deigh-Hewertson, 1978). A word of warning seems appropriate here. Inevitably it will be easier to develop criteria for physical conditions, where measurement is often so easy, and to disregard psychological conditions, especially where social factors are prominent, where the data are soft and not easily measured. Whilst not denying in any way the need for excellence in physical diagnosis and treatment, it would be dangerous and retrogressive to focus exclusively on this aspect. For years we have fought for the recognition of the holistic nature of general family practice which makes it so different from other disciplines, and now this is recognized. It is essential therefore that our criteria audit is also holistic and that psychological and social factors are subject to audit as well as physical factors.

Assessing what is occurring in practice

Having established the criteria, the next step is to assess to what extent these are being met in practice. In hospitals, trained analysts review the medical records to obtain evidence of meeting or not meeting the criteria. As mentioned earlier, in the community based practice, clinic or health centre, other methods could be used as well, such as observation, case review and discussion. However, it must be conceded that the medical record is the best documentary evidence that is available and, if accurately kept, is the most reliable indicator of what the health care professional actually did. If this is to be the main data source for criteria audit, the importance of good records is obvious. Perhaps criteria audit may become one of the most cogent reasons for upgrading contemporary medical records.

Evaluating whether the criteria are being met

The medical record analyst keeps an account of the percentage of cases where the various criteria are being met and withdraws those records where the criteria have not been met. Providing the records are well kept, this step should constitute no difficulty in community based practice. In analysing the records, the analyst comments on whether unrealistic standards were being set and whether the variations from the set criteria were justified or not justified. In the latter case, remedial action is indicated. He also looks for patterns of deficiencies and their causes.

AUDIT CRITERIA FOR IRON DEFICIENCY ANAEMIA

	CRITERIA	%	EXCEPTIONS	INSTRUCTIONS AND DEFINITIONS FOR DATA RETRIEVAL
JUSTIFICATION	**Diagnosis**			
	1. Haemoglobin (Hgb) < 10 gm%; and	100	1A. None	
	2a. Hypochromic, microcytic cells; or· b. Serum iron < 50 μg% and total iron-binding capacity (TIBC) > 350 μg	100	2A. Absence of iron in bone marrow	2. Hypochromic, microcytic cells = peripheral blood, smear report or report of cell indices for mean corpuscular Hgb concentration < 30% and mean corpuscular volume < 75 cu μ.
	Surgery/Special Diagnostic or Therapeutic Procedures			
	3. Bone marrow aspiration	0	3A. Serum iron > 50 μg%	
	4. Packed red blood cell transfusion	0	4A. Hgb < 5 gm% on admission or congestive heart failure documented	4A. Congestive heart failure = check both physician's progress notes and x-rays for pulmonary or peripheral oedema, basilar rates, ventricular gallop, and third heart sound.
	5. Whole blood transfusion	0	5A. None	
	Admission			
	6. Justified by the diagnosis	100	6A. Presence of congestive heart failure	6A. See instruction 4A.
OUTCOME	**Discharge Status**			
	7. Satisfactory response to therapy; and	100	7A. None	7. Satisfactory response = Hgb increase of 1.5 gm% over admission level or reticulocyte count increase of 2% over admission level.
	8. Documentation of investigation of etiology of blood loss; and	100	8A. None	8. Investigation = menstrual history and pelvic exam for females. If normal —and for males—stool gualac (Haemocult), sigmoidoscopy, upper gastrointestinal series, and barium enema.
	9. Documentation of plan of management of underlying cause of blood loss	100	9A. None	
	10. **Mortality**	0	10A. None	
INDICATORS	**Length of Stay**			
	11. Minimum: 4 days maximum: 10 days	100	11A. Complications or additional diagnoses extending stay 11B. Patient died before 4th hospital day	11A. Extending stay = documentation in both physician's progress notes and orders of either therapeutic or diagnostic measures regarding a complication or additional diagnosis.
	Complications		**Critical Preventive and Responsive Management**	
	12. Congestive heart failure	0	12A. Packed red blood cell transfusion	12. See instruction 4. Correlate cases not meeting critical management with criterion 4.
	13. Haemolytic transfusion reaction	0	13A. None	13. Haemolytic transfusion reaction = temperature > 101°F, chills, and renal shutdown (< 20 ml urine/hr) or Hgb in serum or urine.

Figure 2 Audit criteria for iron deficiency anaemia. Reproduced with the permission of the Joint Commission on Accreditation of Hospitals

Taking corrective action

If criteria are unjustifiably not being met, corrective action is needed. A remedial educational programme should be developed to correct inadequacies revealed by the audit. This could be done by way of the practice tutorial, by practice clinical meetings or by case review using the group discussion method, or if only one person is concerned, individual instruction or even self-directed study may be all that is necessary. Occasionally, a policy change or administrative reorganization may be the most appropriate action.

Reassessing the effect of corrective action

After corrective action has taken place, it is essential to recheck the situation by repeating the audit at an appropriate time. This follow-up will indicate the success or otherwise of the remedial programme. If deficiencies persist, further remedial action will be needed, and this step repeated until such time as the criteria are being met consistently.

Considerable emphasis has been given to criteria audit in this chapter, although it is seldom used at present in community based practice. As public and political pressure mounts for review of health professional standards, this method promises to be perhaps the most feasible and rewarding for this mode of practice.

WHAT PHYSICAL FACILITIES ARE NEEDED FOR EDUCATION IN THE PRACTICE?

Most of these have been mentioned in the previous pages and so they will simply be listed here.

Minimum requirements are:

1. A room for meetings and group discussion.
2. A quiet library area.
3. Educational equipment such as an audiocassette recorder, a 35mm slide projector, (some units combine these two), an overhead projector and a white or black board.
4. A good medical record system, preferably problem-oriented, and if possible typewritten.

Useful additional, although more expensive facilities include:

1. A video camera, recorder and monitor.
2. One-way mirrors for observing consultations.
3. A computer terminal and storage facilities.

It can be seen that many existing practices either do provide or could provide the minimum equipment with little expense.

WHAT PEOPLE ARE NEEDED FOR EDUCATION IN THE PRACTICE?

The people are more important than the technology. An optimal educational situation will include:

1. Trained supervisors who understand teaching and learning.
2. A mix of allied health professionals in the practice or associated with it.
3. Readily available resource people for tutorials or individual advice or instruction.
4. A cooperative practice staff which encourages educational activities.
5. An informed practice population which recognizes the value of the practice becoming an educational environment for medical personnel at undergraduate, graduate and postgraduate levels, as well as for nursing staff, social workers, other allied health professionals and administrative staff at all levels of training and experience.

What other features are necessary for education?

Perhaps the most important is an efficient and effective system of practice management which enables staff to be involved in educational activities. If properly organized and managed, the practice can provide opportunities for most of the continuing educational needs of the practice staff.

A MODEL FOR THE EDUCATIONAL PROCESS

To conclude this chapter, brief reference will be made to a useful model for the educational process. It is compared with the medical process with which we are all familiar.

The steps in the medical process are:

1. Define the medical problem or diagnosis.
2. Determine the objectives of remedial treatment.
3. Plan and carry out the remedial treatment.
4. Assess the outcome.

The steps in the educational process are similar:

1. Define the educational problem or diagnosis.
2. Determine the objectives of remedial education.
3. Plan and carry out the remedial education.
4. Assess the outcome.

Ways in which these steps can be carried out have been detailed throughout this chapter, especially in the section on professional standards review.

CONCLUSION

It can be seen that there is an abundance of opportunities for education in the practice environment if staff members are willing to seize them. There is little needed in the way of expensive facilities or equipment. Every staff member can be both teacher and learner if he or she wishes.

Thus the practice can richly enhance the other learning activities of the practice staff which are undertaken privately. Books, journals, self assessment programmes and other educational materials will always be available. Their value is established. The educational activities of the practice can bring these materials to life by relating them to the problems of real patients – your patients.

References

1. Fabb, W.E., Heffernan, M.W., Phillips, W.A. and Stone, P. (1976). *Focus on Learning in Family Practice*, pp. 35-46, Melbourne, Family Medicine Programme, Royal Australian College of General Practitioners.
2. Knowles, M. (1975a). *Self-directed Learning*, p. 18, Chicago, Association Press Follett Publishing Company.
3. Knowles, M. (1975b). *op. cit.*, p.9
4. Royal College of General Practitioners (1972). *The Future General Practitioner – Learning and Teaching*, pp. 218-223, London, Published for RCGP by the British Medical Journal.
5. Kagan, N. (1975). *Interpersonal Process Recall: a Method of Influencing Human Interaction*, East Lansing, Michigan State University.
6. Smith, S.R. (1977). Application of the tracer technique in studying quality of care. *The Journal of Family Practice*, **4**, 505-510
7. Byrne, P.S. and Long, B.E.L. (1976). *Doctors Talking to Patients*, London, H.M.S.O.
8. Fabb, W.E. and Marshall, J.R. (1983). *The Nature of General Family Practice*. (Lancaster: MTP Press)
9. Corley, J.B. (1976). *Evaluating Residency Training – an Operational Prototype*, Charleston, S.C., Medical University Press.
10. Fabb, W.E. and Marshall, J.R. (1983). *The Assessment of Clinical Competence in General Family Practice*. (Lancaster: MTP Press)
11. Heffernan, T.M. (1978a). *Programme Evaluation Methodology*, mimeographed document, Melbourne, Family Medicine Programme, RACGP
12. Heffernan, T.M. (1978b). *Administration Methodology*, mimeographed document, Melbourne, Family Medicine Programme, RACGP
13. de Dombal, F.T., Leaper, D.J., Horrocks, J.C., Staniland, J.R. and McCann, A.P. (1974). Human and computer-aided diagnosis of abdominal pain: further report with emphasis on performance of clinicians. *British Medical Journal*, **1**, 376-380
14. Australian Council on Hospital Standards, Australian Hospital Association, Australian Medical Association (1978). *A Guide to Clinical Review – a Manual on Clinical Criteria Auditing*, 1st edition, pp.13-17, Sydney, ACHS, AHA, AMA.
15. Clark, M.R. and Putnam, R.W. (1977). *An Assessment of the Impact of Patient Care Appraisal on Physician Performance in an Ambulatory Setting*, mimeographed grant application, Halifax Dalhousie University.

16. Greenfield, S., Kaplan, S.H., Goldberg, G.A., Nadler, M.A. and Deigh-Hewertson, R. (1978). Physician preference for criteria mapping in medical care evaluation. *The Journal of Family Practice*, **6**, 1079–1086

13
Practising Primary Care in Developing Nations

M.K. RAJAKUMAR (MALAYSIA)

Primary care is both the oldest as well as the newest discipline of medicine. In developing nations, primary care is still a discipline without a name. It is regarded as an adjunct to hospital practice, a necessary evil to the good practice of hospital medicine. Like the man who discovers that what he has been writing all his life is prose, only in recent years has there been an awareness that primary care has always existed as a vital but neglected part of the health services.

The pattern of health care in developing countries has been frozen at the colonial pattern of 20 or 30 years ago. The independent governments have continued to build more and expensive hospitals, lacking an awareness that health needs could be met in any other way. A wealthy urban elite has sustained this trend to meet their personal needs, using specialists as primary physicians for their families.

The situation in developing countries is that four-fifths of the population live in rural areas but four-fifths of all doctors are in the urban areas. Four-fifths of morbidity and mortality are in the rural areas but four-fifths of health funding goes to the urban areas. Four-fifths of health problems need primary health care but four-fifths of the health budget goes into hospitals.

The task in these countries is two-fold. Firstly, recognition must be won for the importance of primary care and its relevance to the health of the nation. Secondly, standards of practice must be raised so that the excellence of its practitioners becomes obvious.

The people to do this are the traditional general practitioners. They are usually part of the elite of developing nations, often children of influential families, and their own children may be specialists in hospital practice or in the administrative elite. Nevertheless they are closest to the community and sensitive to its needs.

They practice, however, under extremely diverse conditions. At one end you may have isolated rural practices with solitary physicians who receive no journals and attend no refresher courses, practising intuitive medicine on a population that cannot afford anything but the cheapest of medicines and

230

investigations. At the other end of the spectrum, you have large medical groups looking after the wealthy urban elite and the foreign expatriates. These groups have all the advantages of practice in the advanced nations, have a stable of specialists at their call and maintain telephone contact with advanced centres in developed countries to refer their patients.

FORMING A COLLEGE

The challenge is to give this diverse group of general practitioners a sense of common interest and common purpose. A college or academy of general practitioners provides such a focus.

Since only a handful of developing nations have colleges or academies of general practitioners, a few remarks on formation may be useful here.

From the outset it must be clear that the college is principally if not exclusively an educational body. Medical politics is for the national medical association in which general practitioners will be adequately represented.

A group is needed to plan and sponsor the college. A period of a year at least must be taken to form this group and to publicize its plans. From the outset the group must undertake educational activities to stress the academic nature of its plans. Weekly or fortnightly educational meetings will quickly separate the sheep from the goats. This original group will be the founder members of the college. When the projected number of sponsors from representative centres have been collected into the group, plans to form the college can be announced.

When the college is formed, work must start on preparing for an examination in two or three years' time. In the interval, alternative methods of entry to the membership should be provided by participation in continuing education and by writing commentaries or dissertations.

The college or academy is a way of pooling expertise. Doctors have many talents and expert groups can be formed around selected members with special knowledge or skills. Different aspects of practice management can be allotted to small groups of two to five persons to study and make recommendations. The other chapters in this book can provide a basis both to aspire to, as well as to improve upon and make relevant to, the distinctive needs of differing societies.

An important management objective is to upgrade the practice by providing continuity of care. The existence of a medical record system is visible evidence to the patient of your commitment to his continuing care. Two other practical measures are patient education and an appointment system. Health education and staff training will also be touched upon, as will formation of groups and research. Finally the place of rural health centres is discussed.

MEDICAL RECORD SYSTEM

One of the top priorities is a system of medical records that is acceptable to the majority of practitioners inside the college for a start. The A4 folder, excellent though it is, is not acceptable on grounds of costs and space as well as being unsuited to the predominantly episodic nature of much general practice in a developing nation.

To introduce a simple system where there is no system at all is a great step forward. Often there are just scraps of paper or serial records in a volume. The first step is to design a simple and economic system that will meet the elementary objective of retrievable records, providing for continuity of record-keeping and a problem orientation.

The idea of the problem-oriented record was first introduced by Lawrence Weed in 1968 in an article entitled 'Medical Records that Guide and Teach' which appeared in the *New England Journal of Medicine*. These ideas were expanded in a book *The Medical Record, Medical Education and Patient Care* first published in 1969.

The problem-oriented medical record (POMR) provides a framework of logical thinking in diagnosis and treatment because it asks the physician to itemize the problems in each patient and to make a formal decision regarding the management of each of these problems. The POMR enables another doctor to swiftly grasp the problems in the patients he takes over and enables a team to participate efficiently in the treatment.

One simple system is described below. It is a transitional system preparing the physician for adopting a full A4 based system later. I call it the Abbreviated Problem-Oriented Medical Record System.

The heart of the problem-oriented system is the identification and formal listing of problems. The card that I am proposing introduces this essential element into general practice records. I am assuming that the majority of practitioners in developing nations are not prepared at this stage to undertake the expense and the extra work of a full problem-oriented system.

The abbreviated system will entail the introduction of a single A6 or a 6" × 4" card as a Basic Data Card into the records of every 'regular patient'. The low cost of this step makes it feasible for practices in which a great number of patients seek episodic treatment.

Explanatory notes

Patient profile

The patient profile is an impressionistic record giving an assessment of the patient's temperament, habits, social and economic situation, and other data that are of value in management in general practice.

Problem list

All problems affecting the patient should be listed and identified by a number. The description of the problem is refined as information becomes available. Under 'status', the problem is described as active or inactive. If

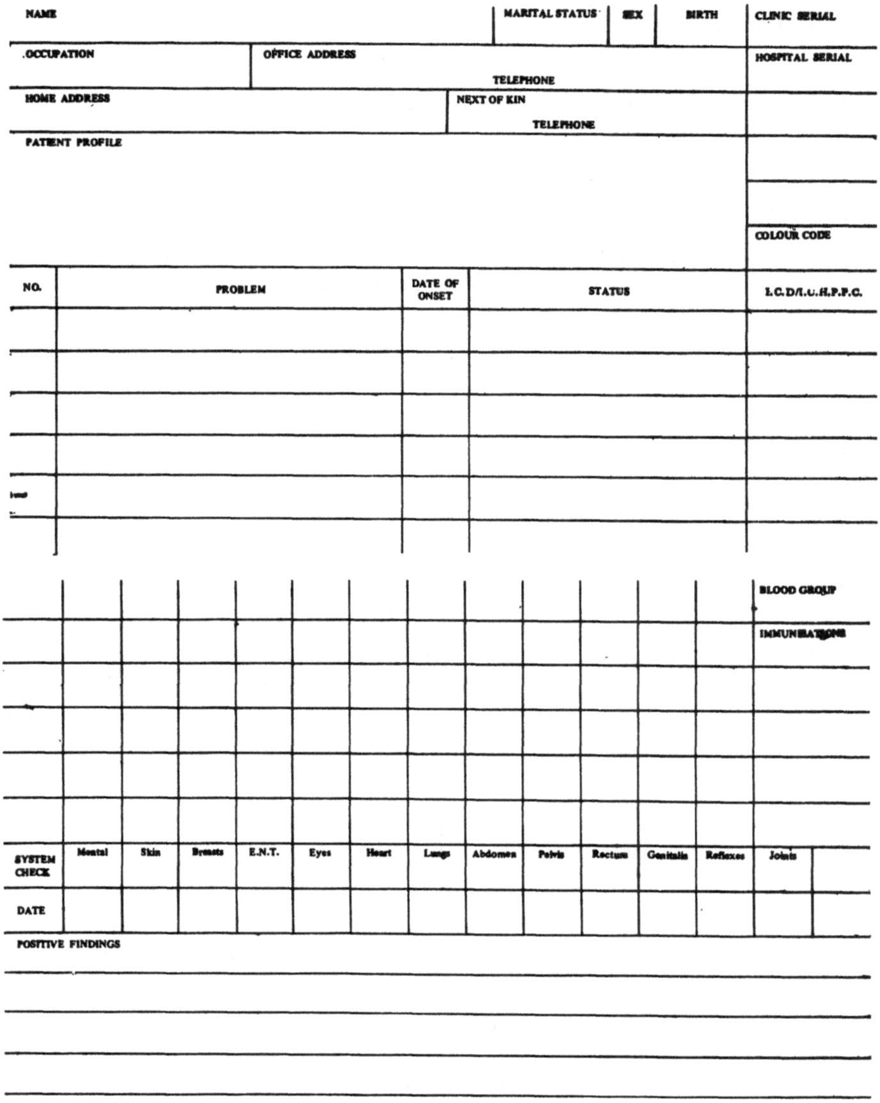

Figure 1   The Basic Data Card

resolved, the date is noted or the dates of recurrence are noted. All significant past illnesses are recorded here.

Colour code

The colour code identifies major illnesses. The Royal College of General Practitioners, United Kingdom uses seven colours to indicate various conditions.

ICHPPC/ICD codes

Spaces are provided for the insertion of a code number according to the ICHPPC or ICD codes. This is done if the practitioner wishes to obtain statistics about his practice.

Flow chart

The space on the reverse of the card enables serial recording of vital data over a period of years. The data selected will depend upon the patient's specific requirements. A separate flow sheet of the same dimensions can be added.

System check

This is an aid to the memory to ensure that over a number of visits spread over a period of time the patient will receive a comprehensive check.

Progress notes

Progress notes are divided into two parts in the customary manner. One column is for subjective and objective findings and the other column is for assessment and plans corresponding to the traditional 'findings' and 'treatment' respectively. The progress notes can be supplemented with flow sheets for frequent recording of selected parameters.

Findings Subjective–Objective	Treatment Assessment–Plans

The next step that the practitioner could take would be to record his findings under each numerically identified problem. The treatment of each problem would similarly be identified.

The system that I have described is a very basic one serving as an introduction to the problem-oriented system. It will enable the practitioner to cultivate the habits that go with the problem-oriented approach, and to discover for himself how valuable it is to himself, educationally and functionally, as well as to the welfare of his patients.

AN APPOINTMENT SYSTEM

This is discussed elsewhere in this volume but if you are not willing to implement those excellent ideas, try a minimal appointment system. A minimal system only asks the patient to come back on a certain day, perhaps specifying morning or evening.

An appointment for a specified day will increase patient compliance. It answers two questions in the patient's mind, that you **want** to see them again, and that you thing it is **important** for them to come again. By giving them a card and writing down the date of the next appointment, you have communicated this. If the patient is asked to bring the balance of the medicine with them, you can check on compliance. Initially it is worth seeing chronic cases more often so that you can check on compliance, provide reassurance on side-effects, and continue education on the patient's role in his own care.

The next advance is to keep a record of appointments and to note those who fail to keep them. Cases where the consequences may be serious to the patient should be given priority for follow-up reminders. In most developing countries, no official machinery exists to help the doctor. He will have to develop his own. Messages can be sent through members of the family, relatives or friends and sometimes by letter. Bear in mind that your erstwhile patient may have moved on to another practitioner, or is happy in the hands of a lay healer.

PATIENT EDUCATION

Even well-educated persons may be ignorant of their own body or of disease processes. The simplest information may be welcome to the patient. Never underestimate ignorance, but be guided by your patient's response.

Patient education cannot be separated into a discrete event. The entire environment must be educational. The walls should project messages on the importance of hygiene, the availability of family planning advice, the advantages of immunization and breast feeding and the dangers of tobacco smoking or driving without seat belts. Patient education should be intertwined into the consultation. Remarks and observations during history taking and examination should prepare the way for more formal advice at the end of the consultation.

By seeking a consultation, the patient has asked for help. The duty of the physician is to communicate to the patient that the most important part of the help he is offering is not the pills, but the information and advice that he offers.

Posters and leaflets should supplement the advice and information offered personally by the physician and his staff. Posters may be available from the Ministry of Health. Simple posters can be designed. Patients may contribute posters. Each picture and phrase must be suited to the culture and socioeconomic conditions of the population to which it is addressed.

Leaflets can be cheaply produced if they are on a single sheet. Small numbers can even be handwritten. A small slip attached to the appointment card can remind the mother of the importance of bringing baby for immunization. A rubber stamp can remind of advice to stop smoking.

The staff in every practice can do a great deal in producing material as well as in personally transmitting advice.

STAFF TRAINING

In most countries, the only trained nurses are hospital-trained, and they are few in number. Usually general practitioners recruit untrained staff and let them learn at work.

The staff of a practice are a most important factor in efficient health care delivery. An informal plan of training can produce impressive results in better patient–practice rapport and in compliance to treatment. Teaching can be in the form of observations made during the course of examining patients, passing round books and articles to read, or even marking out parts of manufacturer's literature.

GROUP PRACTICE

Excepting a few group practices in urban centres, solo practice is the rule in developing countries. The big groups are based on 'contracts' that are given out by large companies for the medical care of their staff. There is no national health service or health insurance although the State generally provides free or subsidized treatment in hospitals for the indigent and for employees of the State.

The solo private practitioner lives on the fees of his patients paid directly to him on a sort of fee-for-service basis. These physicians manifest all the individuality and wariness that is characteristic of the independent contractor, working long hours and taking little time off.

These physicians are precisely the ones who will need a group and will benefit most from a group. But they despair of finding a way to work together.

It is usually not possible for these physicians to form groups based on a single practice. However, coming together even whilst practising separately can be advantageous. I propose a hierarchy of steps towards a full partnership.

1. Bulk purchasing of drugs.
2. Referral of patients back to the nearest doctor in the 'group' for follow-up.
3. Employment with a view to partnership of an assistant to cover leave and busy periods.
4. Sessional work in each other's practices.

RESEARCH

This is treated in Chapter 11. Research is not an optional desirable activity, but essential to efficient primary care. You do not know what you are doing unless you do research. Research need not invariably be elaborate and expensive.

Every practice should adopt a minimum programme of research. I suggest some topics.

1. Morbidity. What are the types of illness seen in your practice? What is the distribution by age group and sex?
2. Is there a seasonal variation of illness in your practice? What is the pattern and incidence?
3. Is there any uncommon types or presentations of disease that you see in your practice? Make a study of this.
4. Is there any geographic distribution of any disease? Chart it on a map and keep track of variations.

Once a college or academy exists, these reports can be published and joint projects involving several practitioners can be organized.

VOCATIONAL TRAINING IN PRIMARY CARE

In a developing country, private medicine is beyond the reach of the vast majority of people. The hospitals are maintained by the State and training in the traditional specialities is provided in them. Invariably there is no formal training and no career prospects for general practitioners in the Ministries of Health.

If primary care is to fulfil the challenging tasks it faces in the developing countries, it needs training centres. It is necessary to lobby for the creation of teaching health centres with the sort of priority for funds that is usually given to teaching hospitals. These centres are especially needed in the rural areas. With the advantage of adequate financing, the health centre can train a new generation of undergraduates and specialists in primary

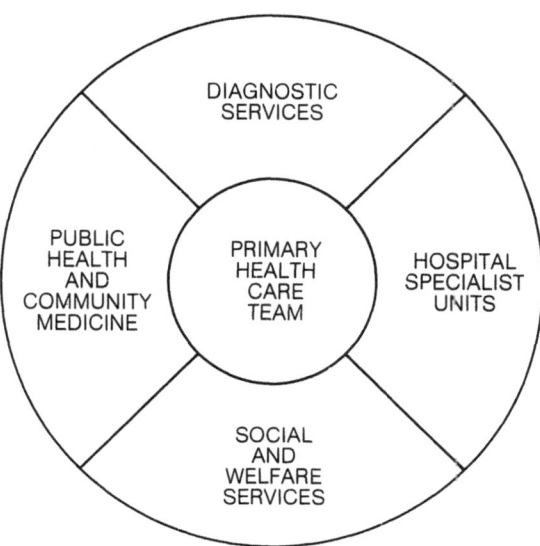

Figure 2   A model for health services

health care. Many of the advanced ideas described in other chapters of this book can then be meaningfully applied at these teaching centres which will serve as a model for other health centres, just as teaching hospitals serve as a model for other hospitals.

This will not come easily. Policy makers will have to be educated. Prejudices that have been unquestioned will have to be subjected to criticism. The accepted pyramidal model of the health services portrays the hospitals at the apex providing, 'advanced and sophisticated' treatment and primary care at the base providing 'basic' treatment of 'simple' illness, overlapping with paramedics and lay healers. Instead primary health care should be presented as the central axis of the health services with hospital specialities filling but one segment (see Figure 2).

CONCLUSION

Good practice management is essential in order to practise efficiently. Ultimately the individual and the family being cared for are the beneficiaries. It is good practice management to take small practical steps rather than to endeavour to implement the impossible. Instead of giving up in the face of difficulties in implementing the innumerable good ideas in this book, study them and invent a simple variant that can meet your needs.

Index